Exhale

LISSETTE RODRIGUEZ

Exhale

A LIFELINE FOR THE LIFE GIVERS

31 Day Devotional for Caregivers

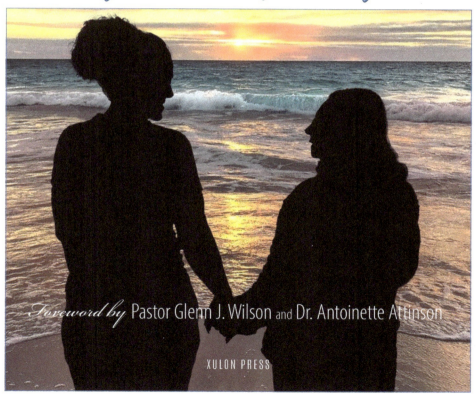

Foreword by Pastor Glenn J. Wilson and Dr. Antoinette Attinson

XULON PRESS

Xulon Press
2301 Lucien Way #415
Maitland, FL 32751
407.339.4217
www.xulonpress.com

© 2022 by LISSETTE RODRIGUEZ

Forewords by Glenn J. Rev. Wilson, and Dr. Antoinette Attinson

All rights reserved solely by the author. The author guarantees all contents are original and do not infringe upon the legal rights of any other person or work. No part of this book may be reproduced in any form without the permission of the author.

Due to the changing nature of the Internet, if there are any web addresses, links, or URLs included in this manuscript, these may have been altered and may no longer be accessible. The views and opinions shared in this book belong solely to the author and do not necessarily reflect those of the publisher. The publisher therefore disclaims responsibility for the views or opinions expressed within the work.

Unless otherwise indicated,Scripture quotations taken from the Holy Bible, New International Version (NIV). Copyright © 1973, 1978, 1984, 2011 by Biblica, Inc.™. Used by permission. All rights reserved.

Paperback ISBN-13: 978-1-66285-296-1
Ebook ISBN-13: 978-1-66285-297-8

TABLE OF CONTENTS

Day 1 – The Beginning: Because they A.G.E.: Already Given Enough. 1

Day 2 – Drawing Strength from the Past: For the days I am weak. 4

Day 3 – Chosen for this Moment: Loneliness. 9

Day 4 – Today is a New Day: Hope. 12

Day 5 – Yeah, You Did That: Stress. 16

Day 6 – Recharge Yourself: Affirmation. 20

Day 7 – Joy for the Future: Faith. 24

Day 8 – Infused from Above: Strength. 27

Day 9 – Today Was a Bad Day: Hurt. 32

Day 10 – Rest in Your Memories: Love. 37

Day 11 – Discomfort vs Regret: Your Rights! 41

Day 12 – The Value of "Me Time": Self-Care. 45

Day 13 – My Safe Zone: Peace. 51

Day 14 – EXHALE: Patience. 55

Day 15 – The Promise: Find Joy. 60

Day 16 – The Golden Rule: Trust. 80

Day 17 – Who Me? Yes You!: Anger. 83

Day 18 – Fatigued But Not Surrendered. 87

Day 19 – Time Management - Time. 80

Day 20 – Today Great, Tomorrow Who Knows: Sovereignty! 97

Day 21 – Don't Judge Me: Doubt. 100

Day 22 – Understanding: I Still Love You. 106

Day 23 – Determined: I Will Love You Till The End. 111

Day 24 – Ambiguous Mourning: Accepting and Mourning. 115

Day 25 – Confidence: Your Love Has Taught Me Well! 119

Day 26 – I Have Rights: I Have Feelings Too! 122

Day 27 – Memories: I Miss Who You Used to Be. 126

Day 28 – FEAR: Can I Really Do This? 129

Day 29 – Anxiety. 134

Day 30 – My Assignment. 138

Day 31 – Until Then. 141

31 Day Devotional for Caregivers

Requirements of a "caregiver" A person who serves with empathy and loves you beyond your abilities to do for yourself."

<u>**Why God chose you**</u> - First let me say, "You're welcome!" The fact that you were chosen is a gift. From birth God chose you and equipped you for the task. Every step you took, every situation you faced, every fall you endured was preparing you for such a time as this. Those situations that seemed to defeat you were really strengthening you for what was to come. Every crisis, challenge, defeat and at times surrender wasn't the end of one thing; but in essence, the beginning of another. Those moments were the ones that defined you and strengthened you in areas perhaps you never even noticed. These situations and moments have made you who you are today! Your worst days have equipped you for your best days! Today, many envy you, dislike you, hate you, misunderstand you, and some even love you because of who you are; however, they would never imagine the cost! There's a high price to pay for being YOU because of your value! You matter!

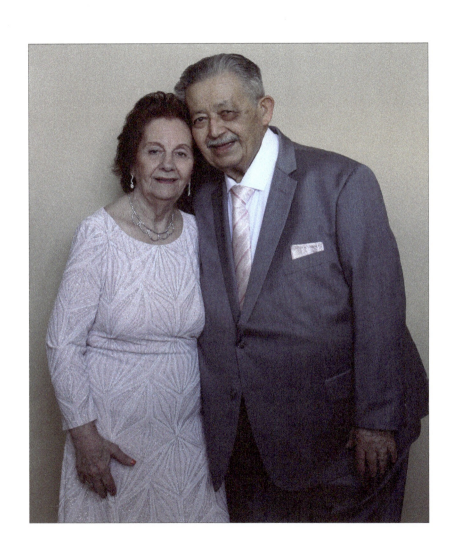

DEDICATION:

To my amazing parents to whom I owe everything!

I would not have experienced the growth nor the inspiration if it weren't for you. Today, I'm here as a better wife, mother, daughter, sister, pastor, and friend because of all that you have instilled in me.

Thank you for well-equipping me for this journey; had it not been for your guidance, unfailing love, and wisdom, I wouldn't be the woman I am today.

I feel so honored to know that God hand-picked me for the task of being your caregiver. Mom, dementia will not rob you of all your memories, for I will continue to remind you and love you just the same. Dad, as your body weakens, I will be your strength. Although this road has not been easy, I wouldn't trade it for the world. You guys have been my rock and my strength, and now it's time for me to be yours.

Thank you for building me on the foundation of Christ. That has been my greatest gift, one that I have been able to impart into my own children. You are leaving such a great legacy. I am able to serve at a greater level because of the strong foundation you built in me. My verbal declaration for you both has been and continues to be, "your last days will be your best days." I pray this has been your experience thus far and will continue to be until the end of time!

Love you beyond words, Lissette

SPECIAL THANKS:

It's A Family Affair

To my amazing husband and children:

There aren't enough words to describe my love and gratitude for you.

Everything I do is because of you! Your help and support have enabled me to become a better daughter and caregiver to my parents. With your help, we are simultaneously fulfilling Gods Promise in Ephesians 6:2-3. THANK YOU for all that you do! I'll forever be indebted to you! I LOVE YOU WITH EVERY BREATH I BREATHE!

To my Overseer and Pastor Glenn J. Wilson:

Thank you for believing in me and not allowing me to quit the task at hand.

Your persistence was key in this development. Your heart for others encouraged me to finish. Thank you for pushing me onward!

To my Mentor Dr. Antoinette Attinson:

Thank you for your spiritual nourishment and guidance. Your wisdom and discernment helped me believe while your love and encouragement paved the way.

PURPOSE

What you're about to read is more than just a devotional, it's a real-life guide through a caregiver's experience. It was written with intent for you to better understand the needs of others. Jesus himself came with the intent to serve others; but we don't understand the cost and sacrifice of serving others until we start to serve. Jesus himself stated, *"Even the Son of man came not to be served but to serve, and to give his life as a ransom for many"* (Matthew 20:28).

As you embark throughout the pages of this daily devotional, it is my heart's desire that it would help you understand the blessing and hardship in serving. It isn't the easiest thing you will ever do; but it will be the most rewarding. The Apostle Paul reminds us not to grow weary in well-doing; for in due season, we will also reap if we do not give up! So, I want to encourage you, if you're actively a caregiver or serving in any capacity, keep up the good work! You are well-equipped for the task. Blessings are on their way!

FOREWORD

Stories very often recount past events; journals mostly extract the day-to-day and real-time happenings in the life of the writer. This journal is a window that gives us access into the widely unknown life of a caregiver.

The author, Lissette Rodriguez, who now accepts this role as a calling from God, will take us on a moment-by-moment narrative of the highs and lows, tears and joys, fears and courage, stress, and rewards of this assignment.

As she shares her experience, you will arrive at the conclusion that sometimes God asks us to step out into the great unknown; there, He teaches us things that we could've never learned otherwise. It's from that place that the author, Lissette Rodriguez, opens the door and lets us into the experience of the journey on which she was sovereignly placed.

This book, like no other, will take you into the inner chambers of the unpredictable life of a caregiver, from the lowest and the darkest moments of this assignment to the joy of loving those who first loved us; and it will provide a daily path to help you EXHALE.

To those who are currently caring for a loved one who is battling dementia or any other disease that incapacitates them and renders them totally dependent on your care, get ready to receive a daily dose of strength and encouragement. Ultimately, you will rediscover the joy of serving those who first served you, and develop the faith and the courage to help you EXHALE with every sunset.

I am honored to have had a front row seat in the journey of faith and caregiving of the author, Lissette Rodriguez.

Glenn J. Wilson
Senior Pastor of Restoration Family Worship Center
Howell, New Jersey

When asked to write this foreword, I was delighted to hear that this devotional was created with caregivers in mind. We often focus on those who are sick, and unfortunately, overlook the struggles of those who care for them. In a world where many will not give without compensation or reward, it is refreshing and life-giving to see love on display during times of difficulty. This devotional is Pastor Lissette Rodriguez' story.

When Pastor Lissette first shared that she would be providing care for both of her parents, she was excited to have the opportunity to love them in this special way. As her journey continued, she realized this love would have to navigate through strenuous exertion, exhaustion, fearful nights, and painful decisions. Grace and love girded her during this journey.

Pastor Lissette shares from a place of experience, how caregiving is a labor of love. This expression of voluntary love does not come without physical and emotional strain, and spiritual depletion. It is my hope that those who read this devotional will be encouraged as they are reminded of the biblical truth found in,

1 Thessalonians 1:3, *"We remember before our God and Father your work produced by faith, your labor prompted by love, and your endurance inspired by hope in our Lord Jess Christ."*

Rev. Dr. Antoinette Attinson,
Christ Church of Howell

A Lifeline for the life givers

Disclaimer: A bad day in the care of my loved ones could never erase the lifetime of love I have received from them.

While I have not earned a medical degree or certification in dementia care; I've earned my title as a caregiver, through my mistakes, experience, and research. Although there is currently no cure for dementia and medications only provide a delay of progression, my prayers and faith have provided me the strength and courage needed to continue this journey! In every stage, we will all experience similarities in situations; but our ways of handling them will be unique to our Loved One (LO). I would highly recommend following up with your doctor on how to proceed with your Loved One's (LO's) needs since no two people are the same.

My Commitment, Mom your dementia won't stop me! Dad your medical needs can't stop me!

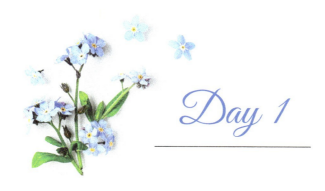

Day 1

THE BEGINNING:

Because they A.G.E.: Already Given Enough

1 Thessalonians 5:18; Psalm 118:24; Ephesians 1:16, 5:20; Acts 24:3

My heart is full of gratitude:

> **1 Thessalonians 5:18** "give thanks in all circumstances; for this is God's will for you in Christ Jesus."

> **Psalm 118:24** "The Lord has done it this very day; let us rejoice Today and be glad."

> **Ephesians 1:16** "I have not stopped giving thanks for you, remembering you in my prayers."

> **Ephesians 5:20** "always giving thanks to God the Father for everything, in the name of our Lord Jesus Christ."

> **Acts 24:3** "in every way and everywhere we accept this with all gratitude."

They often say there's always a way to view a situation. Either your cup is half full or half empty. The way you view a situation will indicate your reaction and outcome. Despite the daily roller coaster of emotions I must confront, I choose to remember the facts of my life! My LO raised me to the best of her ability. She gave me things that money couldn't buy like unconditional love and support. Her hugs were my safe place while her voice gave me peace. I remember that even when I was sick, all I needed was her voice to feel better. It was medicine to my soul. Although I wasn't rich growing up, I was extremely wealthy! While I'm on this roller coaster ride of emotions, I choose to grab ahold of gratitude!

Mom; I make a conscious effort to appreciate all you have already given; and express appreciation to you in returned kindness. Thank you for never giving up: you hung in when things were hard; you never quit and always believed in me; you never left me behind but always pushed me forward; you never cursed me but always blessed me; you never lost faith and always challenged me to believe; you never doubted me but always pushed me to my next. Thank you for seeing things in me that I couldn't see; for giving me all that you had and withholding nothing! You had the chance to give up on me and you chose not to. So Today, I chose not to give up on you because you already have given enough! I'm forever indebted to you! I LOVE YOU MOM!

Father God, Today I pray that whoever is reading this now, You would give them the revelation to see that their cup is half full, it was never empty! That from the beginning of time, You prepared them and equipped them for such a time as this. Throughout their life You gave them a heart full of love, patience, and kindness. You allowed them to experience it so they can be it. Thank you, Father God, for allowing us to now see You were with us all along. I now know I can do this. THANK YOU! In Jesus' name, Amen!

JOURNAL

_____

_____

_____

_____

_____

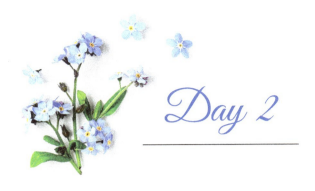

Drawing Strength from the Past - For the days I am weak.

1 Thessalonians 5:11; John 16:33; 1 Peter 5:10; Philippians 4:13

> **1 Thessalonians 5:11** "Therefore encourage one another and build each other up, just as in fact you are doing."
>
> **John 16:33** "I have told you these things, so that in me you may have peace. In this world you will have trouble. But take heart! I have overcome the world."
>
> **1 Peter 5:10** "God always gives you all the grace you need. So you will only have to suffer for a little while. Then God himself will build you up again. He will make you strong and steady. And he has chosen you to share in his eternal glory because you belong to Christ."
>
> **Philippians 4:13** "I can do all this by the power of Christ. He gives me strength."

Who knew we would be living through a pandemic? It has taught us to live life intentionally and carefully. Another day is never promised to anyone, so while I'm here, I would like to fulfill my God-given assignment before leaving this earth. I want to believe that my life will impact and somehow bless someone else's life. I strongly believe that we were created with a purpose, for a purpose, on purpose; so today, I will just sit back and go down memory lane, with hopes of recognizing some of the tools I was handed to draw strength for living.

In hindsight, one of the greatest things that has impacted my life is the level of faith my LO demonstrated. Faith is a word that requires action. You not only declare the things that are not as though they were, as the Apostle Paul wrote; but you believe that they already are by acting on them. I saw this time and time again as I watched my LO pray at her bedside nightly. Although nothing seemed to change in the natural, the next day she would walk with such confidence and authority as if it already was. The look of fear she had would leave once she prayed. Eventually, I would be a witness to things turning around in our favor or others' petitions being answered. I witnessed this time and time again. As I watch her live out her life of faith, I am strengthened by what I observe with my very own eyes. Her faith soon became my faith!

I saw her use her faith in action as she prayed over people and situations. I saw God move in our midst as she preached and taught God's word. I came to know God through her level of faith in Him. Faith was something you saw in her and desired to have.

Some things you learn from others by observing; and I'm blessed that my LO imparted into my life using both methods.

Another tool my LO used and still uses till this day is prayer. I watch as she prays and receives strength, confirmation, and answers. Even now with being at stage 5-6 of dementia, when I ask her to pray, she prays with such conviction and power. At times, I open my eyes and stare at her as I listen intently to her prayers. There's just something about a praying mother that touches God's heart. When we go to church, I observe her worshiping God as if dementia doesn't exist in that moment, only her faith.

Another tool my LO used and uses till this day is worship. I watch her raise her hands and speak praise and adoration to her living, powerful God. I saw how her circumstances would change, her mindset would change and ultimately her life. She would always tell me, "Lissette in times of trouble, worship will get you through, never underestimate the power of worship!" I never knew back then that she would be imparting to me for my now. I am forever grateful.

Father, I just want to say in the midst of all my doubts, thank you for reminding me of the tools I already have for what I'm facing. I took time to look back at life and now I see how You have well-equipped me. I have tools like faith, prayer, and worship! I've seen them operate and work in the past, so please give me the strength to use what I've been given and see the fruits of it once again. I hope you are well-pleased in all I do. In Jesus name, Amen!

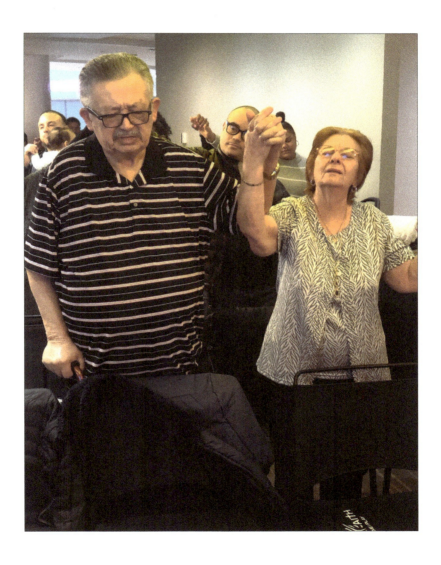

JOURNAL

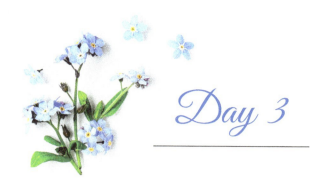

Day 3

Chosen For this Moment: Loneliness - The ability to feel alone even when surrounded by others.

John 14:18; Joshua 1:5; Psalm 25:16; Psalm 62:8

John 14:18 "I will not leave you as orphans; I will come to you."

Joshua 1:5 "Just as I was with Moses, so I will be with you. I will not leave you or forsake you."

Psalm 25:16 "Turn to me and be gracious to me, for I am lonely and afflicted."

Psalm 62:8 "Trust in him at all times, you people; pour out your heart to him; for God is our refuge."

Loneliness can be an overwhelming feeling of isolation regardless of where you are and who's around. It's often the lack of an emotion being met from a need you're having. It can also be described as a "no time for me" feeling. Although these feelings are very real, we need to come to the understanding that these feelings are only indicators; and should never become dictators. When you look at something as an "indicator" it'll help you take your next step in the right direction to fulfill your needs. The greatest mistake we can make while feeling "lonely" is to continue to compound the feeling by looking to blame others without truly assessing the root of the issue. While blaming others can seem like the right answer, it couldn't be farther from the truth. I know you may be thinking "Why me?" "Why do I have to do this alone with so many other people around?" Because You Have Been Chosen For The Task!! I have a little secret to tell you.... while at times you want to quit, you're tired, angry, and frustrated, the Truth Is... You have been chosen because no-one can do it like you!!!! There, I said it!!! In the midst of these struggles, determine to find the strength in looking for the solution that will eventually solve your issue of feeling lonely. If you STILL feel lonely while being surrounded by others, then it's a clear indication that the answer is within bursting to come forth. So Today, I challenge you to look in the mirror and confront the very thing that is causing you to feel "lonely." By understanding the root of your feelings, you can then understand the "why" you're feeling like that. If at some point, our LO met one of our emotional needs, then evidently, we will have to face the feeling of loneliness once they are no longer able to fulfill that emotion. However, now the challenge will be in finding a positive way to deal with the lack of what once was. Are you ready to look in the mirror and confront this? I need you to think before you react!

Father, help me make the hard decision of choosing to look at myself first. In my anger and frustration, help me see that the answer is in me not them. I trust You knew what You were doing when You chose me for this task; but there are times I still question why. I don't know how long I will have to endure; but whatever time it is, I trust You already have a plan in place, and it will all work out in the end. Please guide and lead me every step of the way and whatever You do don't let go of me!! I can't do this on my own. Thank you! In Jesus name, Amen!

JOURNAL

_____

_____

_____

_____

_____

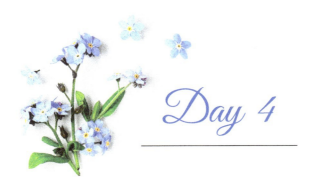

Day 4

Today is a New Day: HOPE - The ability to still believe

Jeremiah 29:11; Romans 15:13; Romans 8:24-25

Jeremiah 29:11 "For I know the plans I have for you," declares the Lord, "plans to prosper you and not to harm you, plans to give you hope and a future."

Romans 15:13 "May the God of hope fill you with all joy and peace as you trust in him, so that you may overflow with hope by the power of the Holy Spirit."

Romans 8:24-25 "For in this hope we were saved. But hope that is seen is no hope at all. Who hopes for what they already have? **25** But if we hope for what we do not yet have, we wait for it patiently."

The reality is that NO ONE understands your struggles like you do. No one can ever speak to you from a position of understanding unless they're on your same journey. This, at times, is so frustrating that it makes us lose all hope.

Yesterday was such a hard day. It started early in the morning when my LO refused to take her meds (as she often does). She hid them under her tongue then tried to convince me she had taken them. I saw her looking for a napkin, and while she said she wanted to wipe her mouth; I knew she was getting ready to spit them out. When I confronted her, she got angry and she literally shoved me out of her way, then screamed, "You can all go to hell because I'm leaving for good." She walked into the kitchen and stared out the door with such a lost look on her face. I stood 10 feet behind her just watching to make sure she didn't leave, while all along asking myself, "where's my mom?" She would have never!!! Minutes later, she went into a full-blown anxiety attack. She started crying and apologizing for her actions. It was almost like my mom came back for a few minutes to apologize for what the imposter did in her absence. Instead of being angry or resentful, I put my feelings and thoughts aside to reassure her while she's crying and apologizing. For that moment, my feelings and emotions didn't matter because she was first; but it was so hard not to cry along with her. I literally felt like a ticking time bomb that needed to be contained because that was not what she needed. She needed reassurance and comfort which only I could give while my own heart was breaking. I wasn't mad at her; I was just hurt and needed my mom while I was trying to be her's. Talk about role reversal! The one thing I will say is that EVERYTHING I'm able to do Today is because of all the love she gave me growing up.

Today I cried and was so hurt; but being able to give my mom back a little bit of what she gave me all my life made me grateful and hopeful. I don't know what tomorrow will bring; but I choose to grab ahold of HOPE! Life is full of choices, options, and emotions we can live out. While depression, anger, frustration, bitterness, resentment, anxiety, and fear want to take residence in my life, I CHOOSE HOPE! It's a choice we must make daily. The Psalmist said it best, "Oh Lord, for what do I wait? My Hope is in You!" (Psalm 39:7).

Father God, Today I repeat the words of your prophet Isaiah, "But they that wait on the Lord shall renew their strength; they shall mount up with wings as eagles; they shall run and not be weary, and they shall walk and not faint!" (Isaiah 40:31). Although I don't understand why I'm going through this, I made a choice to grab hold of Your strength when mine is gone, Your joy when mine is nowhere to be found and Your peace in the middle of my storm! Thank You for keeping me thus far. Truth be told, I don't know where I would be on this journey without You. Thank You for being there every step of the way even on days I want to quit. You gave me the gift of HOPE! Love you Lord, Amen!

JOURNAL

_____

_____

_____

_____

_____

_____

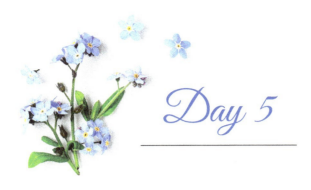

Day 5

Yeah, You Did That: Stress – Your response to pressure

James 1:2-4; John 10:10; Romans 3:23; 2 Corinthians 5:17

> **James 1:2-4** "Consider it pure joy, my brothers and sisters, that whenever you face trials of many kinds, **3** because you know that the testing of your faith produces perseverance. **4** Let perseverance finish its work so that you may be mature and complete, not lacking anything."

> **John 10:10** "The thief comes only to steal and kill and destroy; I have come that they may have life and have it more abundantly."

> **Romans 3:23** "for all have sinned and fall short of the glory of God"

> **2 Corinthians 5:17** "Therefore, if anyone is in Christ, the new creation has come: The old has gone, the new is here!"

In being a caregiver, you will inevitably experience some level of stress. Although we can all handle stress differently, it's definitely part of this journey. Stress is never something we choose; but in doing the necessary, it can become part of the package.

The problem in picking up and doing the necessary is we don't factor in what we already have accumulated on our plates. Our plate called "life" is already so packed with things we chose, that when we need to do the necessary, we become overwhelmed, and it leads us to stress.

I prayed for years that I would be able to care for my parents in their old age; and I'll be honest, I had no idea what I was asking for. I really had no clue how hard, stressful, and challenging it would be. Maybe that's why God took years before granting me my heart's desire. I never took into account that I was already a daughter, wife, mother, professional, pastor, leader, motivator, mentor, and friend to mention a few. In wanting to be my best at everything I love to do, I encountered stress. I was beyond overwhelmed and falling into depression. Everything I had to do required a big part of me serving; and in prioritizing, I discovered that they were all priority, hence the stress. How do I give everything my undivided attention and all of me? I'm on an emotional roller coaster. I'm snapping at everyone because I'm angry, fed up and distressed while smiling and serving, all in trying to keep everyone happy and things in order. I finally discovered that putting myself first was the answer!!! Once I was at my best, they all received the best from me. I became intentional about working on myself first! I know that sounds selfish, but I discovered it worked! I woke up and went to the gym at 5am. I was able to release unwanted stress and worries. I soon realized that on my way back home to take care of my parents and family, I was happy, in a good mood, and energetic. At times I felt like I could take on the world. Although it was a huge sacrifice waking up so early and going to the gym when I mentally didn't want to, I soon discovered it was exactly what I needed. Nothing good comes without paying a price and investing in yourself. During the first few months of the pandemic, I lost 43 lbs. and felt great, not to mention I had so much more energy to do what I was called to. Did you catch that? Yes, I realized I was "called" to do this! It was one of my God-given assignments and it became so clear. It actually brought joy to me to know that God trusted me with such a task! Growing up, my parents gave me the best life they possibly could and now it was my turn to make sure their last days were their best days! So, what I'm saying is that stress was only an indicator that there was more in me which I had yet to discover. I never knew I had this type of strength within me. Take a moment and think about all you do for your LO. You are amazing, strong, loving, patient, and caring – it takes so much to be YOU! It took stress to point it out to me that I was built for this! I may have lost my temper a few times and made a few mistakes along the way; but now I see it was just the tool God used to make the best ME! Sometimes we don't know what we have within until crisis reveals it. Today, I challenge you to take stress and allow it to reveal your strengths! It's easy to focus on the negative; but can you allow stress to point out your strengths?

Father, I thank You for allowing me to see that stress is simply an indicator that I need to focus on my strengths. I didn't see it at first and I need you to forgive me for my short temper, my attitude, my hurtful words at times, and my anger towards others and You. You have been there all along even when I felt alone. Thank You for not leaving; but showing me I had everything I needed because You loved me enough to equip me for the task. Please help us all see that You're always there and that there's purpose for our pain. I now see it as a blessing, and I love You for it. In Jesus name, Amen!

JOURNAL

_____

_____

_____

_____

_____

_____

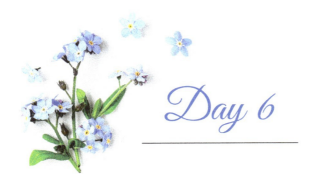

Day 6

Recharge Yourself: Affirmation - A positive assertion

2 Timothy 1:7; 1 Peter 2:9; Philippians 4:13; Deuteronomy 31:8

> **2 Timothy 1:7** "For God hath not given us the spirit of fear; but of power, and of love, and of a sound mind."
>
> **1 Peter 2:9** "But you are a chosen people, a royal priesthood, a holy nation, God's special possession, that you may declare the praises of him who called you out of darkness into his wonderful light."
>
> **Philippians 4:13** "I can do all things through Christ who strengthens me."
>
> **Deuteronomy 31:8** "The Lord himself goes before you and will be with you; he will never leave you nor forsake you. Do not be afraid; do not be discouraged."

In the position of caregiver, the demand and expectations are so great that, at times if we're unable to fulfill a task, it's so easy to feel like a failure! You must make it a point to remember although you're not perfect and you can't be everywhere, at the same time, you're still handling a task that many can't handle.

Remember all you have already done! Against all odds with no training, you managed to take care of your LO when everyone else said, "no!" I remember the day my father finally agreed to move in with me and my family. I say, "my father," because although my mother was with him, she was already in the latter stages of dementia and he no longer had the ability to care for her with all his medical ailments; not to mention he was already 82 yrs. old. While they lived in another state and I already had my own family to care for, I accepted the challenge. This meant going to Florida while my home was in New Jersey, selling their home and packing up 20 years worth of memories and furnishings. What a task!! I had no idea what I was in for; but I embraced the journey and got it done with the help of some of my siblings.

If you're reading this and you are or have been a caregiver, then you already know we never really know what's next. Everyone's journey is different in many ways, yet the same. What an oxymoron.

I intentionally bring to memory all I have already accomplished in hopes of encouraging myself for what lies ahead. No one can affirm me like I can affirm myself. No one knows the cost of this journey unless they have paid the price to walk it. While many can't see all I have accomplished, my experience has paved the way to a satisfaction of which only I would know the value. While others can criticize me or cast judgment, it doesn't devalue who I am or what I've done. Remember that value is placed by the manufacturer and not the consumer.

So Today, I encourage you to remember you have what it takes to walk down this road. If you can't affirm yourself, I want to personally affirm you. The very fact that you even tried is a great deal!

Be intentional and remind yourself how far you've come! Be intentional and treat yourself to a dinner, movie, massage, manicure, pedicure, or just a car ride by the water. If you don't have anyone around to encourage you, then be intentional and encourage yourself. You got this! Just recharge every now and then and keep on going! I'm rooting for you!

Father, I ask that You somehow give us the recharge and affirmation we need to continue down this road. Be our strength when we feel weak. Be our comfort in the middle of the storm. We know its been Your grace that has carried us thus far. In trying to be our best for our LO, remind us that we need to recharge ourselves too. Give us wisdom and strategies for what lies ahead in Jesus' name! Amen.

JOURNAL

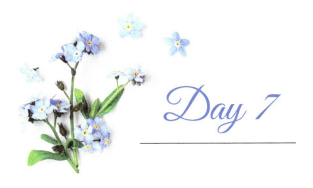

Day 7

Joy for the Future: Faith – The ability to believe in the unseen

Matthew 21:22; Hebrews 11:1-3; 2 Corinthians 5:7

> **Matthew 21:22** "If you believe, you will receive whatever you ask for in prayer."
>
> **Hebrew 11:1-3** "Now faith is confidence in what we hope for and assurance about what we do not see. **2** This is what the ancients were commended for. **3** By faith we understand that the universe was formed at God's command, so that what is seen was not made out of what was visible."
>
> **2 Corinthians 5:7** "for we walk by faith, not by sight."

Choosing joy for the future is an intentional action.

I know you're probably asking yourself right now, "why in the world would I choose joy? There seems to be no end to this heartbreaking journey. Joy is the last thing I can see in my future." Because letting go of the things we can't control and having compassion for others including yourself is a choice!

Too often we neglect the gift of joy by thinking we have to earn it, or it has to be given to us; but JOY is a gift we give ourselves. Joy is a choice! You are intentionally shifting your focus away from your problems and hardships while thinking about the needs of others. It gives you a new perspective in life. It allows you to see the bigger picture. "That can actually be you, but it's not!" You could have lost your mind and despite how you feel, the truth is you haven't. You are still in your right mind and have the ability to make choices! When choosing, choose JOY!

Joy is a decision that goes hand in hand with faith. You're choosing to believe what you cannot see. While we've all experienced different emotions, joy is believing that everything is going to be ok despite (fill in the blank). We don't allow our circumstances to determine how we feel or believe; but we choose what we believe and that leads us to how we feel. I believe that in every circumstance that comes our way, if we choose right, we can become better or bitter, stronger or weaker... life is full of choices. It all depends on how you choose to see things.

You will never know how strong you are unless you've been tested. I hated being tested in school; but our teachers didn't test us to be mean, but rather to prove to us that we're smart! You see, you'll never know the strength you have within until you're forced to use it. Life has a way of helping us discover our abilities with every circumstance it throws our way. We just don't realize it until circumstances force us to use the very thing we're unaware of. I know you're angry and you have the right to be BUT look how far you've come? Did you ever think you would be able to do this? Well now you know YOU CAN!! I'm proud of you!

Father, I just want to thank You for allowing life circumstances to mold me and make me stronger. I never knew I had this much strength in me till now. As I ponder about life, this may have not been the path I chose but I'm grateful for it. Truth be told, I would've never known how strong You made me till now. Please continue guiding me in Jesus' name, Amen!

JOURNAL

_____

_____

_____

_____

_____

_____

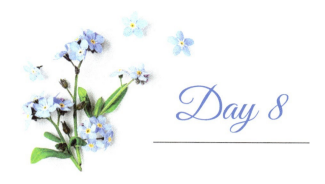

Day 8

Infused From Above: Strength – The ability to withstand great force or pressure.

Ephesians 6:10; Psalms 73:26, 31:24, 29:11

> **Ephesians 6:10** "Finally, be strong in the Lord and in his mighty power."

> **Psalm 73:26** "My flesh and my heart may fail, but God is the strength of my heart and my portion forever."

> **Psalm 31:24** "Be strong and take heart, all you who hope in the Lord!"

> **Psalm 29:11** "May the Lord give strength to his people! May the Lord bless his people with peace!"

These last few weeks have been so hard. It seems to be one thing after another. I noticed my LO's eating had declined. This particular evening, I gave her meds and noticed she was very quiet. I would ask her questions and she would mumble, but then answer. My daughters had made plans to take me to dinner so I left my LO with my father thinking she would be ok. As I arrived at the restaurant and ordered, my phone rang. My sister called me to let me know mom sounded off, she wasn't making sense and her speech was slurred. I left my daughters and ran home to find what my sister had said was true! I got her dressed, struggled to get her to the car because by then she was barely moving so I rushed to the ER, leaving my father behind. The Hospital still wasn't allowing visitors due to this pandemic. How do I split up? I'm the caregiver for both my parents; but I can't be in two places at once. I didn't know how I was to do this all on my own; but I did and somehow, I had the strength needed to accomplish it all. It turns out that mom had a fever affecting her speech. It broke my heart every time I tried to speak to her and she was unable to communicate. She would stare at me with glazed eyes as if she wanted to communicate with me. I was so stressed and worried; but I had to try and reassure her that everything was going to be ok. Well, they ran all types of tests and started an antibiotic through her IV. I was so tired I laid my head on her lap, and she began to stroke my hair. I gently looked up and smiled at her. Suddenly, she smiled back called me by my name and said, "I love you" my eyes weld up with tears. For a minute my mom was back! I saw it in her face! She knew who I was and called me by my name! Suddenly it gave me the strength I needed to keep going!

The doctor decided to admit my LO but allowed me to stay! Throughout the night she never slept. It had now been

21 hours and there was no rest for me in sight; but somehow I had strength to stay up with her and help the nurses care for her. We talked, or should I say I answered her same questions over and over till I lost count! I don't know how I managed to stay up; but somehow, I knew God was giving me the strength I needed to endure. I decided to turn the TV on in hopes of getting her to concentrate on something other than asking me the same questions. While going through the channels, I stopped and focused on a sermon by Priscilla Shirer. She was speaking about this supernatural strength and how God had strategically made her see that she had all she needed to move forward. I felt like that message was just for me! I was strengthened and was ready for my next! I knew at this point, with no sleep for close to 24 hours, that God had to be my source of strength! My sister arrived around 11 am the following morning to relieve me. I went home took care of my dad, fed him, and gave him his meds. I did a few things that needed to get done and went back to the hospital. GOD had become my source of strength.

I know we all have had these types of days. When you're a caregiver you never know what to expect; but we must always be ready. The kind of strength and wisdom we need can only come from above. Have you ever looked back at the end of tough day and asked, "how did I make it through?" Even when we don't acknowledge it, we're infused with strength from above.

Father, Today I've come to the realization that You must have been giving me strength all along. When I look back, You are the only explanation possible. NO one else can do what You have done. Forgive me for not acknowledging You for it. I just want to take this moment to say THANK YOU! You always know exactly what I need even when I don't. I appreciate You being there. Please stay. In Jesus' name, Amen.

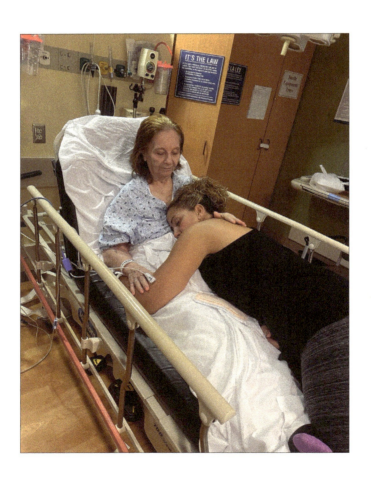

JOURNAL

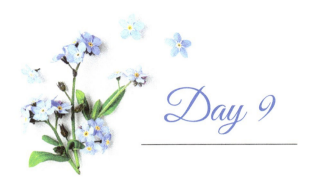

Day 9

Today Was A Bad Day: Hurt

Matthew 11:28-30; Romans 5:3-5; Romans 8:28

> **Matthew 11:28-30** "Come to me, all you who are weary and burdened, and I will give you rest. **29** Take my yoke upon you and learn from me, for I am gentle and humble in heart, and you will find rest for your souls. **30** For my yoke is easy and my burden is light."

> **Romans 5:3-5** "Not only so, but we also glory in our sufferings, because we know that suffering produces perseverance; **4** perseverance, character; and character, hope. **5** And hope does not put us to shame, because God's love has been poured out into our hearts through the Holy Spirit, who has been given to us."

> **Romans 8:28** "And we know that in all things God works for the good of those who love him, who have been called according to his purpose."

After waiting for my parents to move in with me for years, they're finally here! Our first errand was to switch everything over from their previous address to their new address. I knew it would be a hard task due to the pandemic; but never knew it would be a heart breaking one.

A couple of months had passed. I was waiting for the right day and opportunity to present itself. If it wasn't my dad, it was my mom; but usually one of them wasn't feeling well, had an appointment, or my mom was having one of her anxiety attacks as she was trying to acclimate to her new surroundings.

I was finally able to gather all the pertinent documentation needed and it was actually a nice day out. Both of my parents were looking forward to going out. When we arrived at the DMV, I parked right out front. I remember getting out of the driver side and walking all the way around the car to let my parents out. I started to guide them towards the door when I thought to myself, "let me go ahead of them and hold the door open for them." In trying to do what I thought was right, I made the biggest mistake ever! I stood holding the door at the DMV open for them while watching them holding hands and walking together. Suddenly, my LO trips over her own foot. I couldn't believe it! It felt like it was happening in slow motion. I ran towards her to try and catch her, but her face hit the cement sidewalk. She started bleeding profusely as she broke her nose and bruised her face. When I went down to the ground to hold her, she looked at me with this look of terror in her eyes, she was so scared and all she kept on saying was, "I don't know how this happened" almost like she was expecting to get in trouble. I immediately called 911 and tried to stop the bleeding. All I could say was, "mom I'm so sorry!" I felt an immeasurable amount of guilt that consumed me. Here I'm supposed to take care of my LO and she falls in my care. At the same time, I had to calm my dad down, I didn't want him having a heart attack due to the scene.

It felt like the ambulance couldn't arrive fast enough. My mom's glasses had cut her around her eye, and she needed stitches. I just was in disbelief. How did this happen? Why did this happen? The feeling of hurt, pain, and guilt were so overwhelming .

We arrived at the hospital, they took care of mom, stitched her all up, ran all kinds of test and everything went well besides her broken nose. I was worried about internal bleeding since she was on blood thinners; but thank God she was fine. I took her home, comforted her and felt like her mom. I didn't want to leave her side for a second. I started to realize that this task I was looking so forward to was going to be more difficult than I anticipated. However, that didn't scare me as much as the fall did. I didn't know what the future held; but I was determined to become better for her. My pain became a metamorphosis! Whatever happens to you in life allows you to make choices. You can't control what happens, but you can control the outcome of the situation. Let whatever you encounter make you better for the experience instead of bitter. You have the ultimate say in your reaction to the circumstances. So be determined to make it a positive one.

That same night and days to follow, my LO would look in the mirror and say, "I look so ugly, I don't know what happened, look!" And all I could do is reassure her that she was beautiful and that she would heal with time. But if I could be honest, it was a constant reminder of how I failed to keep her safe. I became more and more determined to do better by her because she deserves the very best! I made a decision that day and have honored it to this day!

I want to encourage you; I know you're doing your very best so don't spend time beating yourself up. This journey didn't come with a list of instructions; but it did come with YOU, a person who is willing to try and love your LO in the process! Today, I want to tell you how proud I am of every step you've taken. Even when you've wanted to quit you haven't! You're AMAZING!!! NO ONE CAN DO IT LIKE YOU! So, remember that we're all in this together.

Father, can You please encourage the person reading this right now? There have been some unintended failures; but help them see that You're with them and that You are willing to guide them. I pray that these failures don't consume them, but help them make decisions for a better outcome. Just remind them that You know this task isn't easy so You're willing to equip us with exactly what we need, in Jesus mighty name! Amen!

JOURNAL

_____

_____

_____

_____

_____

_____

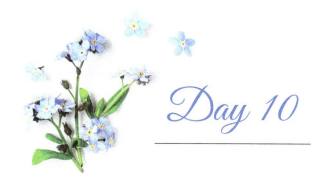

Day 10

Rest In Your Memories: Love

Romans 8:28; 1 Peter 4:8; John 15:13

> **1 Corinthians 13:4-7** "Love is patient, love is kind. It does not envy, it does not boast, it is not proud. **5** It does not dishonor others, it is not self-seeking, it is not easily angered, it keeps no record of wrongs. **6** Love does not delight in evil but rejoices with the truth. **7** It always protects, always trusts, always hopes, always perseveres."

> **1 Peter 4:8** "Above all, love each other deeply, because love covers over a multitude of sins."

> **John 15:13** "Greater love has no one than this: to lay down one's life for one's friends."

It's true what they say, "you never know what you have until you lose it" even though I always appreciated the counsel of my LO and our relationship, I miss it terribly. I never pondered on the thought of her not being present. Although she's still alive and well physically, this horrible disease called dementia has erased her memories and ways of thinking. Due to her dementia, I've had to make decisions on my own. Her counsel and opinion were always the ones that sealed the deal.

When I think back, she had such a hard childhood. Her father took her out of school in third grade to take care of her nine half brothers and sisters. She cooked, cleaned, and would go down to the river to wash everyone's clothes, including her stepmothers' families. In this day and age, she would've been considered a slave. She did all of this at the tender age of nine years old. It's amazing to me that even now she can still read and write with such little schooling.

She never disclosed her childhood to me; but she made sure I knew how to cook, clean, and take care of myself. Whenever we spoke, her wisdom was beyond her years! I just never knew what she had to endure to obtain it. Both she and my father retired to Florida and there was not a day that I wouldn't call just to hear her voice. I remember very well that no matter what circumstances, obstacles, or crisis we confronted, she always faced it straight ahead and her faith in God was immeasurable. Even now, I take her to church on Sundays and she hasn't forgotten how to praise and worship. She still prays with power and conviction. I look at her and just smile. I am who I am Today because of all she, along with my father, has imparted to me.

When I think back on memories of my childhood, I just smile and rest in what once was. Although this horrible disease has affected my LO's memories, I will keep them alive in my heart and thoughts forever! I truly rest in them.

Of course, I could allow the present to rob me by allowing anger, resentment, frustration, bitterness, or loneliness to consume me; but I choose not to! I chose love! This disease has stolen enough! I will rest and take refuge in all she has already given. It's now my turn to give back! We are creating new memories full of love, laughter, and joy! I tell her all the time, "Mom, I know you have forgotten a lot of things; but I'm going to remind you how much I love you, what a great mother you are, how blessed I am to still have you, and how I'll always be here for you." Out of every emotion I can express, I choose LOVE! "And even when you no longer remember me, I'll always love you Mom."

Father, Today I ask that You would give us eyes to see and strength to hold on to that gift of love that covers it all. It covers our pain, frustration, bitterness, and heartache. Love gives us hope and helps us continue down this unknown journey. While anger tries to rule my emotions, please allow love to be stronger and overcome them all! I really need Your help, Lord. Amen!

JOURNAL

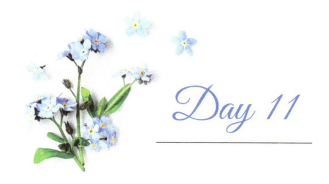

Day 11

Discomfort vs Regret: Your Rights!

John 14:27; 2 Timothy 3:16-17; 1 Thessalonians 5:21; Galatians 6:9

> **John 14:27** "Peace I leave with you; my peace I give you. I do not give to you as the world gives. Do not let your hearts be troubled and do not be afraid."

> **2 Timothy 3:16-17** "All Scripture is God-breathed and is useful for teaching, rebuking, correcting and training in righteousness, **17** so that the servant of God may be thoroughly equipped for every good work."

> **1 Thessalonians 5:21** "but test them all; hold on to what is good"

> **Galatians 6:9** "Let us not become weary in doing good, for at the proper time we will reap a harvest if we do not give up."

So, my life has totally changed in tending to my LO's. I'm 51 years old and I can no longer come and go as I please. My day is surrounded by their needs and wants. Gone are the days when I can just leave on a whim. Their well-being has consumed my every step. Not only have I lost my freedom, but I've gained fear and worry. I haven't slept a whole night since I started taking care of them. I listen to my LO's every breath while they sleep and check in on their moves while I'm out running errands. I tried going on vacation while I left others caring for them; but still found myself concerned and constantly checking in. At night while on vacation, they invaded my dreams. I awoke crying at the thought of not being there physically if something were to happen. Their comfort and care are extremely important to me. Somehow, I'm unable to disengage no matter who stays with them.

I've had to rearrange all my responsibilities and reprioritize according to my LO's needs. I'm unable to work outside of the house because she cannot be left unattended. The freedom I once had is no more. I've become her caregiver, nurse, doctor, driver, chef, secretary, therapist, counselor, accountant, shopper, maid, sounding board, pastor and remain her calm loving daughter. Many often ask, "how do you do it all?" The truth is, I didn't know I had a choice.

While all these functions must be done and require a great amount of sacrifice, I have no regrets. My love and gratefulness towards her supplies me the will to continue.

As hard as life may be at times, I still pray for God to extend her days, even knowing all that entails. I may experience discomfort; but one thing I'm sure of, I'll never experience regret. The satisfaction I will live with after they're gone with the Lord, will bring peace to my heart. It's been a privilege thus far in serving them. These memories are priceless and although they've come with a cost, I thank God for the blessing of being able to serve them. In hindsight, I now see how He has been equipping me all along. Even during the process, I can honestly say He's blessed me with unmeasurable strength and love. I believe I'm better for this experience. I would've never known such selfless love had I not had this experience. Although many emotions at times rock my soul to the core, the faithfulness of God never failed me. While many focus on the anger, bitterness, resentment, frustration, and troubles of the caregiver's experience, I choose to focus on the gift it is! I finally get to give them back a little of the much I received growing up! So, for now I choose the discomfort because regret for me is not an option!

Father, today I grab ahold of Your promise in Deuteronomy 5:16 where it says, "Honor your father and your mother as the Lord God commanded you, that all your days may be long, and that it may go well with you in the land the Lord your God is giving you." Thank You for giving me eyes to see things differently. Thank You for the endurance to run this race! In Jesus' name, Amen!

JOURNAL

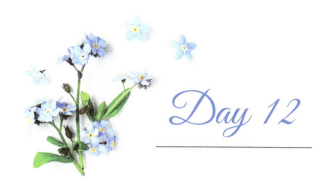

Day 12

The Value of "Me Time": Self-Care

Isaiah 26:3; Mark 6:31; Proverbs 14:30

Isaiah 26:3 "You will keep in perfect peace those whose minds are steadfast, because they trust in you."

Mark 6:31 "Then, because so many people were coming and going that they did not even have a chance to eat, he said to them, 'Come with me by yourselves to a quiet place and get some rest.'"

Proverbs 14:30 "A heart at peace gives life to the body, but envy rots the bones."

I'll admit, at first, I didn't know the value of "me time". All I know is that I started feeling overwhelmed and didn't understand why, because in my mind I was doing what I had to. They were MY parents and I HAD to take care of them because that's what's RIGHT; but in doing what I considered right, I neglected ME! I didn't leave room for self-care at all. What's that? The thought of taking time for myself was selfish of me. My parents needed me. My dad has congestive heart failure, kidney disease, liver disease, a mass on his kidney, hypertension, diabetes, his iron and hemoglobin were low, so I had to take him weekly for either iron infusions or Procrit shots. Since his heart and kidneys aren't functioning properly, I take him once a month for a paracentesis. My mom is suffering from the horrible disease of dementia, so she can't be left unattended and every day I wonder how far she's slipping away. She's fallen numerous amounts of time, even breaking her nose. Here's the problem, I have to push my dad in a wheelchair due to his condition and he's 270 lbs. That being said, it's impossible for me to push him in his chair and guard her as she walks. I try to have her hold on to me, but it's very difficult for her to follow instructions. With that being said, where in the world do I find "me time?" I mean, is that even realistic?

Soon I discovered that I started down a road of depression mixed with frustration and anger. I stopped myself from having emotions too! Every time I felt like I was about to cry, (like when my mom fell on cement pavement and broke her nose) I stopped myself and I remembered thinking, "I don't have time to cry! That's not what she needs!" This soon became my norm, and I just became numb to everything. The only problem was that those close to me started to see my demeanor changing and wondered what was happening. Their questions of, "how are you?" "need anything?" Started to annoy my soul!!! I continued to build this anger unconsciously. I would snap at everything and everyone. It started to affect my relationships all around. I found myself getting angry for not receiving help even though I never asked for it. It was MY responsibility! Anyway, one day I sat with someone I call my second mom. She noticed my change and was concerned. When we spoke, she started asking me certain questions that triggered something inside me. I FINALLY saw that I was so angry at God for everything happening to my mom. The lack of understanding His plan or will was destroying me. You see, my parents were pastors when I was growing up and I grew up in Church all my life. So, I was taught you never get angry at God, you revere Him. I was suppressing all my feelings thinking I had no right to feel what I felt. In conversation with my spiritual mom, she made me see that I had chosen to bottle things up and that's not what God wanted. She got me to see that I was angry at God; I never was willing to acknowledge that until she pointed it out. I remember her telling me, "Baby girl, you can never fix what you're not willing to admit or confront." She gave me a new perspective on what I was experiencing. She made me see that I had to invest in myself and be at my best if I wanted to care for others. Well, I finally broke down and cried. WOW that felt good.... I allowed myself to feel again! She embraced me and I felt like it was my biological mom, I cried and cried. I felt like things were going to be ok again! I guess what they say is true "knowledge is power" because once she made me face my reality, I felt like I could move forward making intentional decisions, even if they came with a price! It took me a while to break that mindset, but once I did, I was FREE! My parents would wake up around 7:30am, so I started to leave the house at 5am going to the gym. At first, I struggled because I felt tired and emotionally exhausted but after a workout, I noticed I felt good and happy. Soon it became a hobby that I still carry till this day. I've had to at times adjust my time frame, but I finally make myself a PRIORITY! It worked!! After a while, as a consequence to my commitment, I noticed the weight loss which in turn boosted my self-confidence and built me emotionally. Today, I make sure I intentionally make time for myself! I go to the gym every morning, that's become my new norm! Sometimes I still struggle with the thought of going but on my way back home I feel great! I serve my parents with a positive outlook and attitude.

They normally go to bed super early, around 6:30pm. So at that point I make plans with my husband and/or kids and I'm intentional about meeting their needs as well. BALANCE IS EVERYTHING!!! Making them happy in turn makes me happy. It is during my "me time" that I have the opportunity to exhale. All the weight we carry in this function as a caregiver has to be released (for me) to walk in peace, love, strength, joy, and freedom!

I never knew that putting myself first, would give those I serve the best version of me! It's a win/win. In being intentional about my "me time", I fully understand that I exhale and exchange all the things I'm carrying for what God wants to pour in me. Ultimately, I found that I'm a better, wife, mother, daughter, friend, pastor, and mentor! Wow, who would've ever known?

Father, Today whoever is reading this, I pray You would enlighten them as You strategically did with me! That You would allow them to understand how putting themselves first is for the best of those they serve. I pray You strengthen them and give them wisdom on how to go about it. I pray that their best days are still ahead, and that joy, peace and love would be their portion now and for years to come. In Jesus' name! Amen!

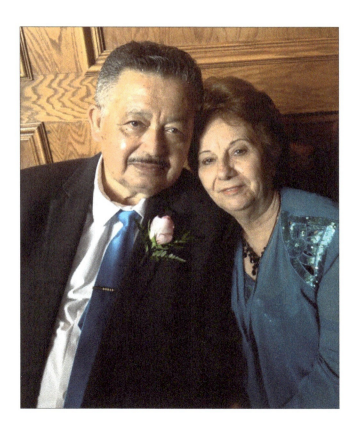

JOURNAL

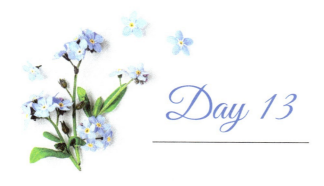

Day 13

My Safe Zone: Peace - Freedom from disturbance; tranquility

Proverbs 18:10; Psalm 91

Proverbs 18:10 "The name of the Lord is a fortified tower; the righteous run to it and are safe."

Psalm 91

Somedays it just seems as if life is a war zone! There's no avoiding it, I just walk through it as best I can. I can't seem to get anything right in the eyes of my LO. From one moment to the next, everything changes, and I am unaware. How did we go from peace to conflict? One second she is laughing and carrying on and the next she is having an anxiety attack. How do I get her to see that what she is thinking isn't true, that her tears and pain are misplaced? There are times she cries for days, and my heart is so broken, yet I must keep it together.

I remember her birthday on June 25, 2021, I had made so many plans to make that day special. I ordered a cake, the family was coming together, we were taking her out to dinner, but she started crying over the loss of her father. No matter what we said or what we planned, she continued to cry in anguish. It was as if it had just transpired now and not 26 years ago. How is she so intensely living in the past? Everyone took off from work to celebrate, but she was too weak to even walk. As she laid in bed inconsolable, she started to cry out to God. I remember seeing her hands stretched out to the heavens as she prayed for God to have mercy! She was so passionate in prayer that I decided to join in. As we prayed, I entered into a place of utter peace! It was like God heard our prayer and His peace fell upon us. I played worship songs on my phone, and I saw her demeanor start to change. She laid there as if she were meditating on the Lord. Some of the songs she even sang along with me. Instantly, all the chaos turned into peace. It was amazing to see that she had not forgotten about the power of GOD! The remembrance of her earthly father brought so much pain, yet the remembrance of our Heavenly Father brought so much peace. It was great to see that all was not forgotten. For a brief moment, she came back! I could tell by the look on her face and the next words she said were, "Lissette I'm so sorry, this is not what I wanted for you." I tried to reassure her of how honored I was to care for her even like this; but just like that, she left again.

In that moment she reminded me of what she had taught me growing up, that in God we have eternal peace. I remembered the scripture she taught me as a child, John

14:27: "Peace I leave with you; my peace I give you. I do not give to you as the world gives. Do not let your hearts be troubled and do not be afraid." Once again in the midst of such chaos she remembered such peace! Even in the midst of this horrible disease she continue to remind me and teach me of Gods faithfulness. These are memories that will hold greater value, due to the circumstances in which they've been taught.

Mom, even in the unpredictable days ahead, due to this horrible disease, you still remind me that the peace of God is sufficient. In God I will always have a safe zone where I can pray, cry for help, scream, share my anger, frustration, and hope without being judged for it. Thank you for the lessons you taught me as a child, they're coming in handy now! I love you mom!

Father, Today was a hard day! Some of us encountered depression, fear, anxiety, anger, bitterness, frustration, confusion, and loneliness along with some tears. Help us find joy in the center of chaos and peace in the midst of craziness we don't even understand. Help us Lord! Some of us took on this task out of love and others out of obligation BUT either way we're doing it and we NEED YOUR STRENGTH WISDOM & GUIDANCE! Give us endurance for the journey ahead. This journey didn't come with instructions but I'm willing to trust You along the way. Tonight, give us rest and please restore all that's been lost. While we take care of our LO, please take care of us, our families and our relationships that are suffering due to the consequences of this journey. The fact that I'm still here is evidence that You're with me, but I need You to intervene on our behalf in Jesus' mighty name! Amen!

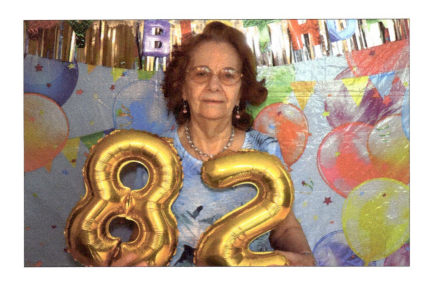

JOURNAL

___
___
___
___
___
___

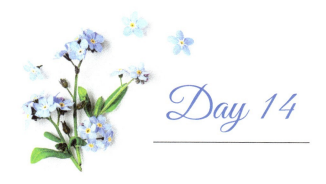

Day 14

EXHALE: Patience - The ability to tolerate or suffer without expressing anger or frustration

Romans 12:12; Galatians 6:9; Ephesians 4:2

> **Romans 12:12** "Be joyful in hope, patient in affliction, faithful in prayer."
>
> **Galatians 6:9** "Let us not become weary in doing good, for at the proper time we will reap a harvest if we do not give up."
>
> **Ephesians 4:2** "Be completely humble and gentle; be patient, bearing with one another in love."

In the beginning when my parents arrived in New Jersey, my father became ill and ended up in the hospital for seven days. I must say, those seemed to be the longest seven days ever. The pandemic had already started so visitation in the hospital was limited.

I remember coming home from the ER where they had decided to admit my dad. My mother was hysterical. I thought she was going to have a nervous breakdown. As I said earlier, they had just arrived in New Jersey from Florida, so I was still in the process of taking them to doctors and setting up visits. I had no medication to give my LO to calm her, so I had to deal with her anxiety attack. After reassuring my LO for hours she finally started to get tired. It reminded me of a crying infant falling asleep. When I finally thought she was resting, she started waking up almost every hour on the hour. I asked her, "mom, where are you going?" She would reply, "I'm looking for your father, I think he's there" I had to repeat myself over and over. This was happening every 1-2 hours. Well, this continued for the next six days, and I had no sleep or help!

I truly struggled, not only with the fact that I was exhausted, but the fear of not waking up in time to stop my LO from leaving! She still did not know my house well enough to maneuver her way around in the dark. What if she fell or left the house? I was consumed with fear. I remember that as each night passed, I was getting angrier at my LO because I was mentally and physically exhausted. It was becoming taxing trying to remain peaceful while anger was grabbing a hold of me. I became angry at my sister for not coming to help and the rest of my immediate family for avoiding the issue all together. Everyone was going about their business; but somehow, I had to figure things out. This was new to all of us, but all of the responsibilities fell in my lap. I was afraid to ask for help, my parents had just arrived, and we were still getting used to having them around. My home wasn't big enough, so my husband offered them our bedroom while we slept in the middle of the family room. Everyone was making adjustments and emotions were high. Everyone had to adjust to a new way of doing things. I couldn't blame my family; if I'm honest I felt so bad for them having to experience such changes. Previous years had been difficult financially and now we finally had our own space, but things changed yet again! I felt like they were my parents, so the responsibility was mine. However, I found myself snapping at my husband and children. I just had a world of anger developing within. While trying to be understanding, I too was suffering the change. Arguments began to arise, but I wasn't focusing on the root, only on the present. I felt the weight of the world on my shoulders, and it didn't seem like anyone realized it. It was the loneliest position to obtain, but it wasn't an option to give up. I still had to be a daughter, wife, mother, sister, pastor, and everything to everyone. Everyone else's needs were being met accept my own.

My LO asked me daily to see my father, so I took her in the wheelchair. At the hospital, visitation was limited to one person per visit per day. I had to explain to the front desk at the hospital that I would only drop her off in my father's room and come back. Thank goodness they allowed it. I had not been gone for one hour when my father would call and tell me to come pick her up because she didn't understand why I left her there, she wouldn't listen to him, and she would wander off. Once again, the anger would build.

I had no downtime at all! I would go pick her up and as soon as we were in the car, she would start crying because she wanted to be with him. It was indescribable! I had to suppress my anger and understand that it was the disease in action. Dementia how much I literally HATE YOU!

Despite the anger, frustration, fear, and exhaustion; that didn't give me an excuse to fall short on my responsibilities. I had to put my feelings and emotions to the side to make sure that everyone else's needs were met.

When dad was finally released and came home, I felt like I could breathe again; but I was still holding in so much anger. You have to be careful that in holding onto anger you don't allow seeds of bitterness to take root in your heart. Once something takes root it's that much harder to uproot. Once a seed is sown it has the possibility of developing into something destructive if left unattended. Once something is left unattended, nothing good can come from it.

You have the right to be angry! Angry at this horrible disease, angry at the loss you're experiencing, angry at the negative changes; but never allow anger to stay planted in your heart. Be intentional on exhaling and releasing every negative emotion! I'm not saying it's not real or that you're not justified in feeling that way; but I am asking that you be intentional in not allowing it to take root in your heart or life.

Remember this disease has stolen enough so don't allow it to steal one more thing from you. Allow your emotions to be indicators and not dictators! Love always wins! So today, choose to exhale and release, it will produce patience while patience produces endurance.

Father, in the name of Jesus, please check our hearts. Don't allow any seeds of anger to stay rooted where it doesn't belong. Sometimes we get lost in our emotions and justifications without even realizing it. Help us be better identifiers than justifiers. We want to have Your heart for others. We need the kind of love that Peter talked about in 1 Peter 4:8 "Love covers a multitude of sins" none of us are perfect. Give us Your eyes to see the truth and Your heart to love the way You love. In Jesus' name, Amen!

JOURNAL

_____

_____

_____

_____

_____

_____

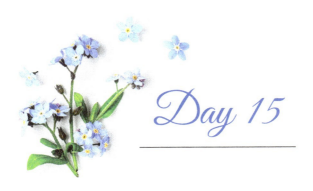

Day 15

The Promise: Find Joy - The ability in finding pleasure and happiness despite what you're facing.

Ephesians 4:2; James 1:2

> **Philippians 4:4** "Rejoice in the Lord always. I will say it again: Rejoice!"

> **James 1:2** "Consider it pure joy, my brothers and sisters, whenever you face trials of many kinds."

Sometimes life hands us unexpected scenarios that don't come with instructions on how to proceed. All we have at times are our past experiences to reference. Every experience comes with a lesson for life. Whether good or bad, it has the potential to mold you into what you will or can become. Who you are Today is the result of what you have experienced.

There are promises we make out of love that can be hard to keep. However, Today I find joy in fulfilling my promise to my mom. All my life she has been the epitome of an amazing woman that is beautiful inside and out, a praying woman, strong, loyal, faithful to the call, full of character and wisdom, always giving, understanding, sympathetic, hardworking, loving, and always had the ability to make the best of every situation. Her wisdom supersedes her age. In my eyes she is the fulfillment of the Proverbs 31 ("The Wife of Noble Character") woman. Today, even as she battles with this horrible disease of dementia, I won't allow it to erase the woman I've always seen growing up.

To my Mother: I can only imagine how hard it must've been raising me. Your love for me was always present. I felt it in the way you held me and protected me. I felt your love in the way you taught me and corrected me. I felt your love when you didn't work just to watch over me. I felt your love when you stayed home to be with me while everyone else went out. I felt your love when you bathed me and dressed me with the clothes you hand made for me. I felt your love when you had patience to teach me right from wrong. I felt your love even when you were willing to repeat yourself so that I wouldn't get it wrong. I felt your love when I was sick, and you didn't leave my side. I felt your love when I made mistakes and you were still there to be my guide. I felt your love even when I disappointed you, but you remained. I felt your love every time I fell, and you picked me up and reassured me I could do it again. I felt your love every time I had a nightmare, and you were there to secure me. I felt your love even after I was married, left home, and moved away. I felt your love in every phone call, post card and visit. Today, even with dementia I still feel your love!

Dementia came without an invite or a warning. Who you once were no longer exists, but my love for you still persists. I promise to say I love you every day just in case you forget. I promise with my actions to display the love you always gave. I promise to hold you by your hand, so you won't feel lost and alone. I promise to guide you every step of the way, so you won't fall or even go astray. I promise to kiss and hug you tight, so you won't forget how much you're loved despite. I promise to dress you like you always liked, so you can continue looking & feeling like your old self. I promise to do what's best for you when you no longer know the difference. I promise to reassure you and make you feel secure when fear knocks on your door. I promise to affirm you when you're confused, and you feel lost. I promise to understand you when anxiety comes and makes you distraught. I promise to dry your every tear when your fears persist. I promise to be patient with you. I promise to keep you from harm's way and protect you. I promise not to let anyone mistreat you because they get frustrated with your ways. I promise to do what's right by you. I'll be your protector. I promise to clean you up and always have you at your best. I promise to be the best of what you need, as you were the best when I was in need. I promise to be the best mom to you as you were to me.

Today, I find joy in fulfilling my promises to you. Although at times I cry because I miss you. The joy I feel at the end of the day supersedes my tears of sorrow and pain.

Father, please help me become everything You've called me to be. Give me the ability to give back all that was given to me, the love, patience, and tender care. If I ever try to give up, remind me of all my LO sacrificed to raise me. You led by example when You gave your best, help me now give back my best. In Jesus' name, Amen!

JOURNAL

_____

_____

_____

_____

_____

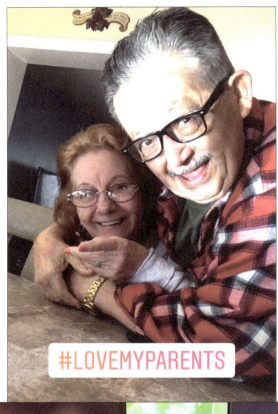
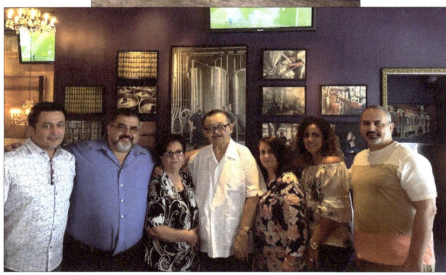

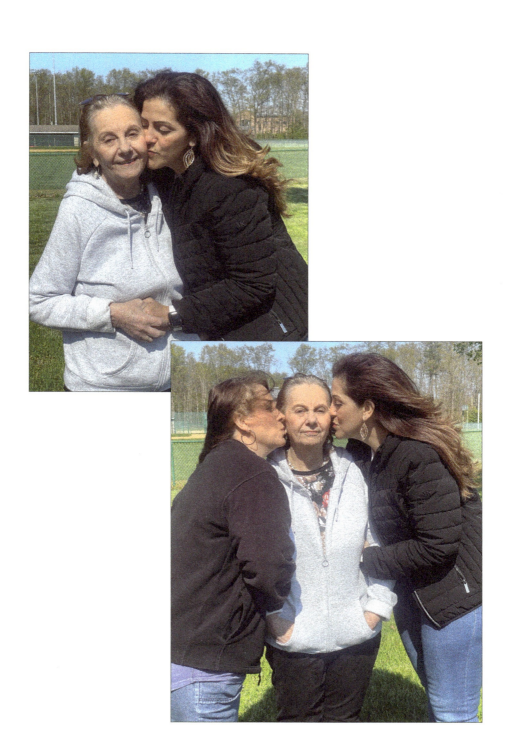

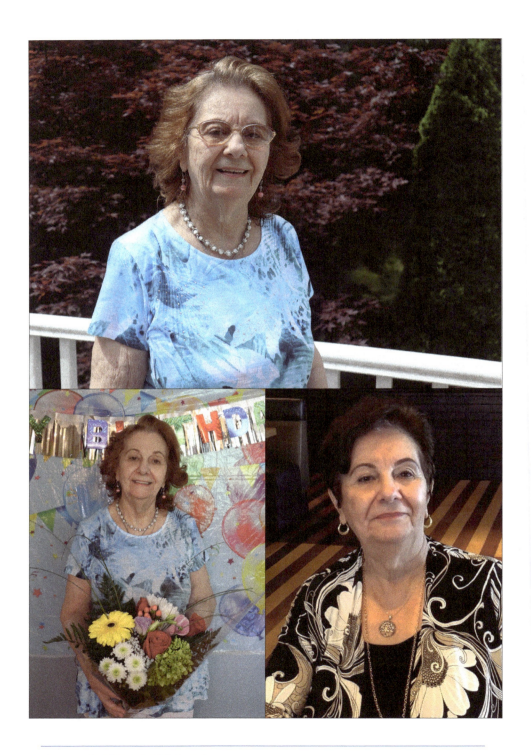

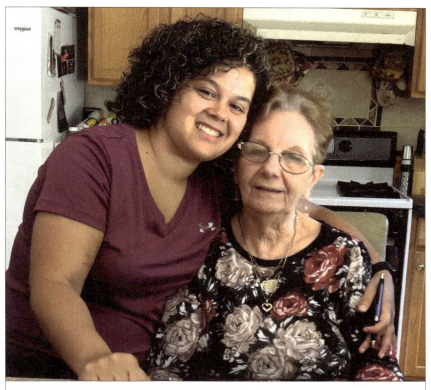

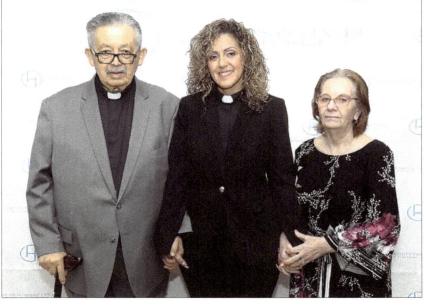

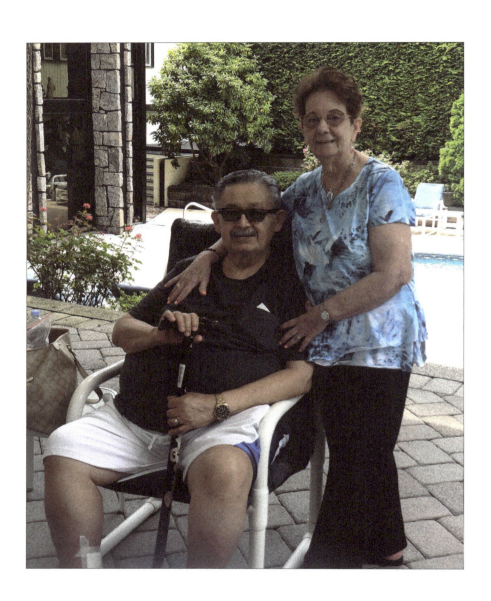

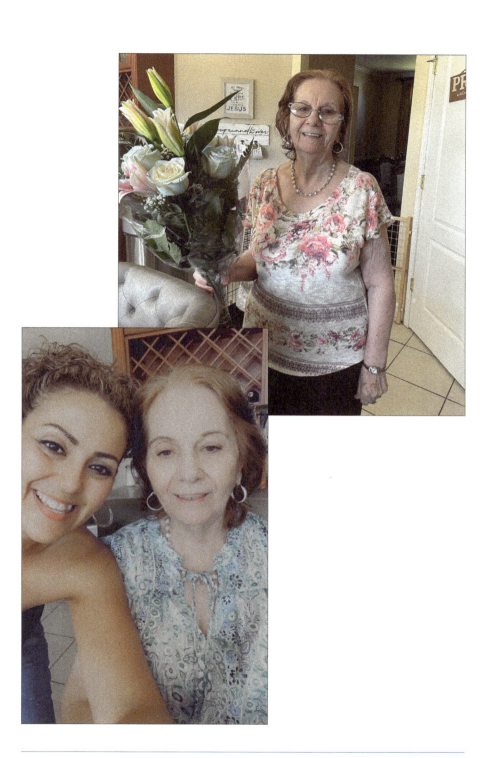

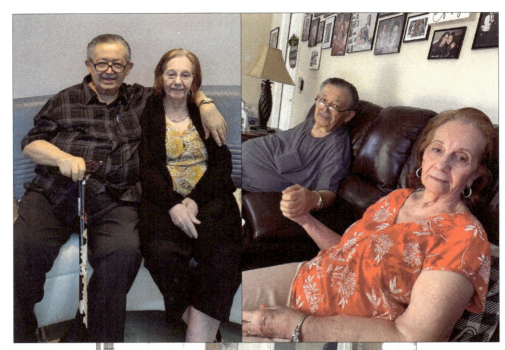
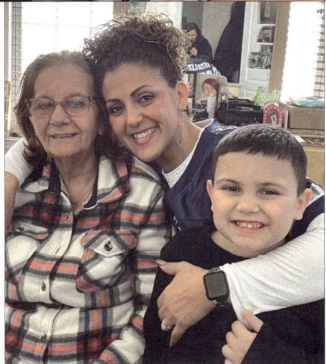

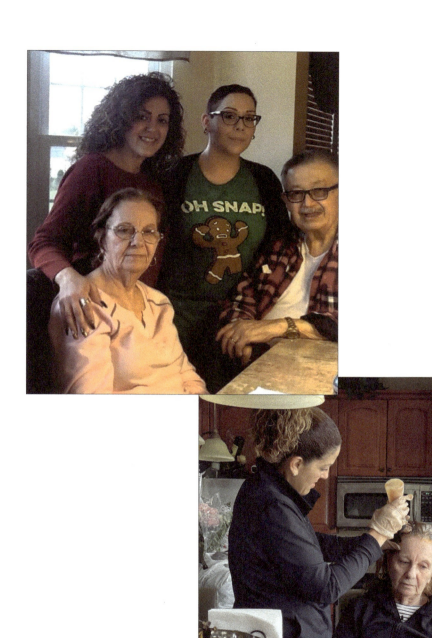

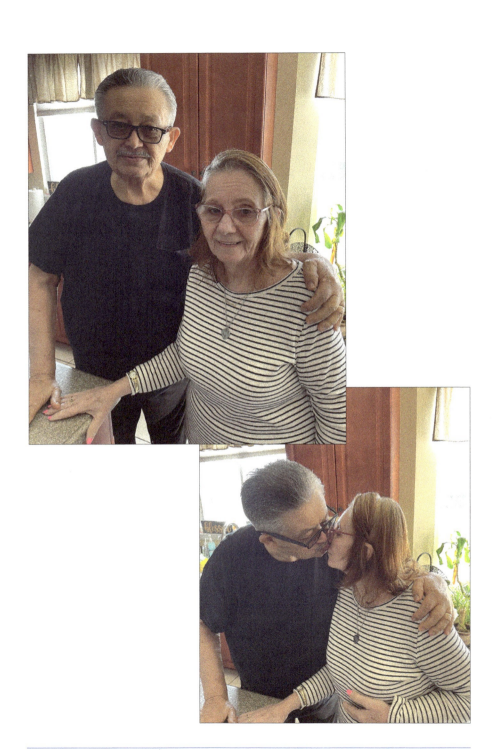

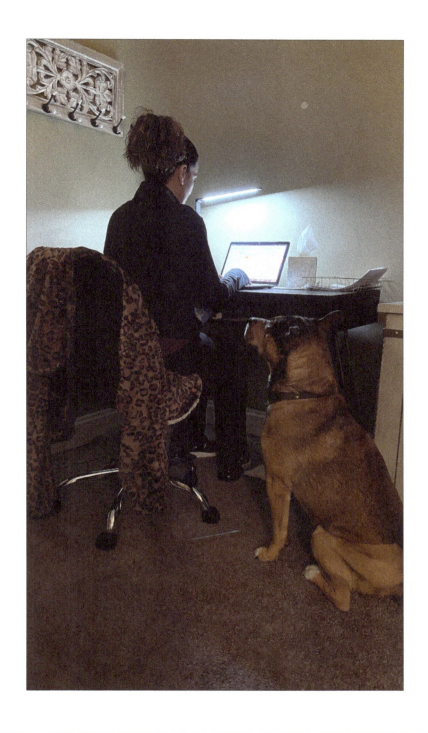

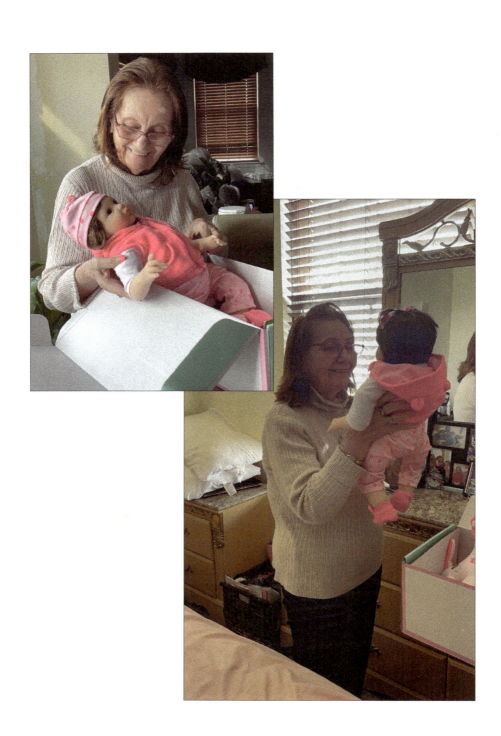

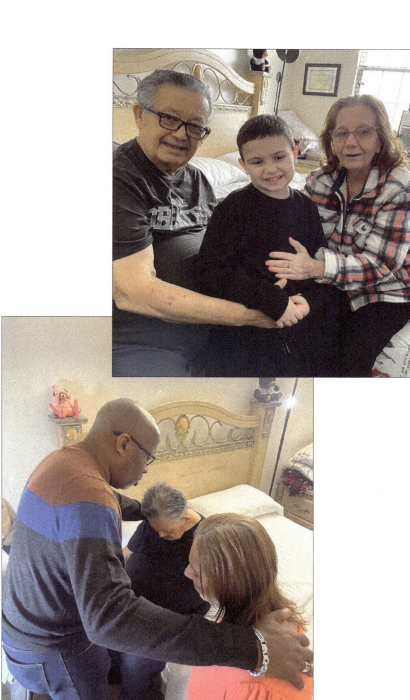

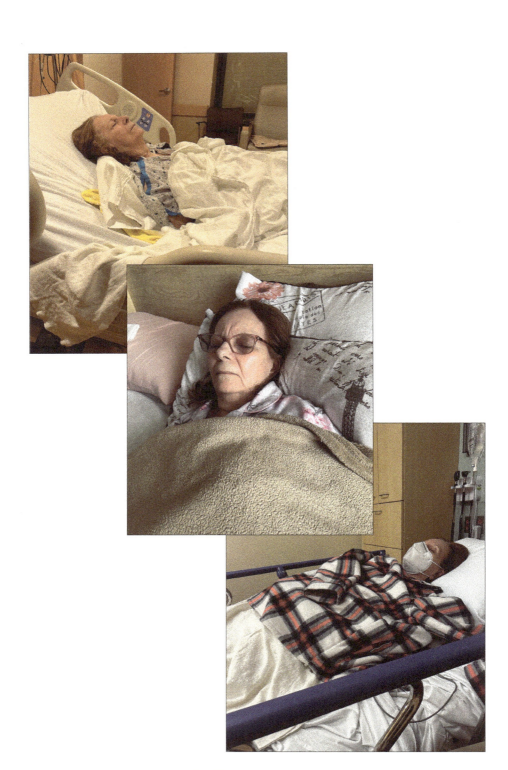

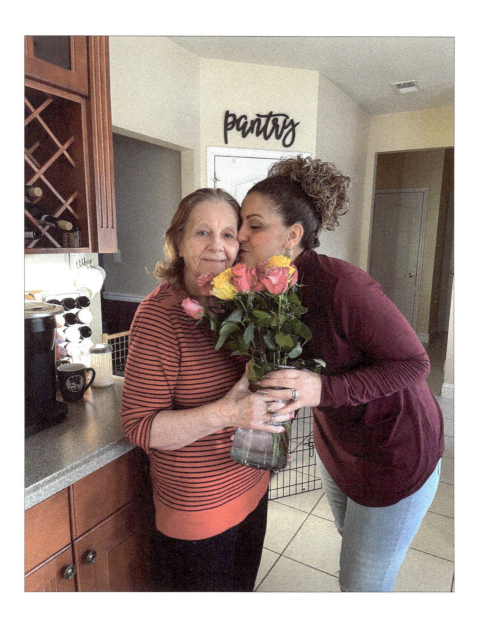

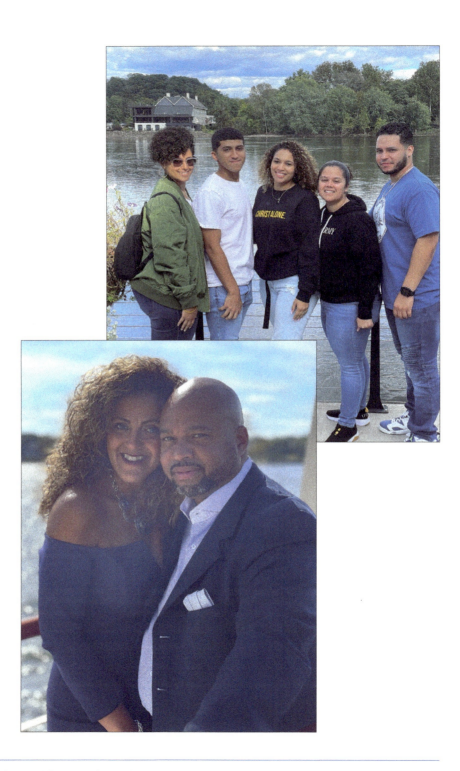

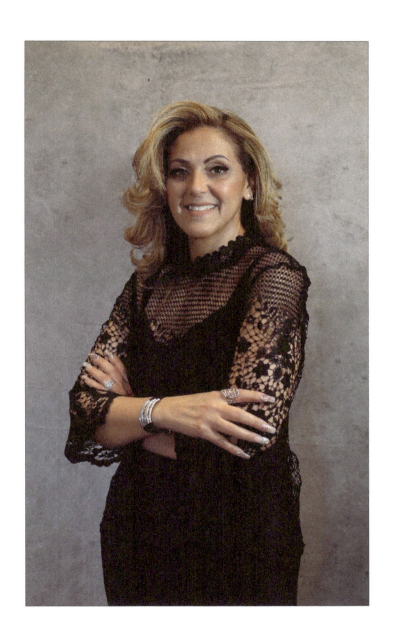

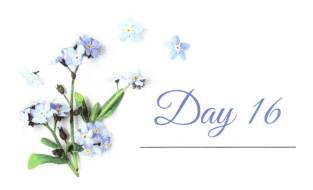

Day 16

The Golden Rule: Trust - Assured reliance on your abilities and strength, the truth of yourself.

Proverbs 3:5; Psalm 9:10; Psalm 56:3

> **Proverbs 3:5** Trust in the Lord with all your heart and lean not on your own understanding.

> **Psalm 9:10** Those who know your name trust in you, for you, Lord, have never forsaken those who seek you.

> **Psalm 56:3** When I am afraid, I put my trust in you.

If you're a caregiver, you will really need the ability to TRUST! First, I want to commend you on stepping up to take the challenge. No one is prepared for this. Every situation is not the same just like every individual is not the same. Today, I came to encourage you to trust what you have within you. While at times you can feel so ill prepared, you're still the best person for the job. Whether you're a daughter, son, niece, nephew, cousin, spouse, grandchild, relative, friend or worker, you obtained this responsibility because no one else could do it like you.

Don't get me wrong, I know all too well that every day is not a walk in the park, but trust yourself. You have what it takes! Take the good days and remember them on the bad days. Trust yourself enough to know you're their best option. You have everything you will ever need within you! Trust your heart is right. Trust they love you enough to be with you. Trust you'll be able to do right by them. Trust that you have made the necessary changes in their best interest.

In the days to come when challenges arise, trust yourself enough to know you'll make it through. When they no longer remember your name, trust they still love you. When they no longer remember who you are, trust they still love you. When they keep you up all night and are restless, trust they still love you. When they see you get angry and frustrated, trust they still love you.

When you feel like you're a total failure because you lashed out, take a break and trust that you're not a failure – you're only human. Your tenacity will help you try again!

When you want to quit and feel like you can't anymore, it's ok, trust you won't. Trust the fact that you have what it takes to do this, and you've been well prepared throughout your life with every obstacle you've had to overcome. All you've endured thus far has well-equipped you for today!

Every day will write its own story and while you're not controlling the dictation, your LO can trust you're the best for the job! It's not about what's thrown at you it's how you react to it. I just need you to trust in yourself and your God given abilities! You are amazing and there's no one like you! Trust that!

Father, help us to trust in who You created us to be. Every time we look in a mirror give us the ability to see You! In You we are strong and more than conquerors. Help us to see and believe we can. Give us the strength this journey requires, in Jesus' mighty name, Amen!

JOURNAL

_____

_____

_____

_____

_____

_____

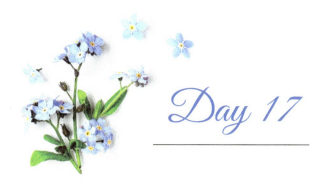

Day 17

Who Me? Yes You!: Anger - the emotion characterized by antagonism toward someone or something you feel has deliberately done you wrong.

James 1:20; Ephesians 4:26; Ecclesiastes 7:9

> **James 1:20** "because human anger does not produce the righteousness that God desires."

> **Ephesians 4:26** "'In your anger do not sin'": Do not let the sun go down while you are still angry,"

> **Ecclesiastes 7:9** "Do not be quickly provoked in your spirit, for anger resides in the lap of fools."

There are times when we experience unexpected circumstances that can be life altering. In refusing to accept these circumstances, many challenges arise, especially at the lack of understanding. The lack of clarity has proven to increase negative emotions, anger being one of many. It's hard to accept something you don't comprehend. The number one question we often have is "Why?" Why my LO, why Dementia? It's such a cruel and horrible disease, it hits everyone differently. While no one has truly mastered the how or why of this disease, it expresses itself differently in everyone, causing different emotions to surface. One minute they're happy and the next angry; one minute they're sweet the next they're mean, you never know what to expect or how your day will be. It's definitely the land of the unknown and that's where many of us struggle.

I remember one particular visit to my parents' home in FL. One morning I was getting ready to go for a walk as I often did, and my LO tells me, "I need you to move out of that bedroom because your sister is coming to visit, and I want her to have the bigger room." I just stood quiet – I think because I was in shock. She had never done such a thing. I visited quite often and even had personal items in that guest room that I had permanently left there. As I went on my walk, all I could do was think about it and anger started to arise, but I also felt hurt. I was staying in the same room I always stayed in, what's the difference now? Why would she do this? Well, when I returned my father was waiting, he noticed the look on my face when I left, and he sat in the garage to wait for my return. When I finally returned, he asked, "Lissette are you okay?" I just burst into tears. I was so full of anger and hurt, my mind was all over the place. I was trying to blame the disease, but I was truly in my feelings. My LO came out and asked why I was crying, and as I started to explain how I felt, she exploded in anger. The words that came out of her mouth were piercing to my soul. I got so angry, but even more hurt. She ended the conversation by telling me how selfish I was and not to bother going to her funeral because she wouldn't want me there. I was beyond crushed. Here I am visiting her from NJ and she basically threw me out! I had to sit in the room and remember that no matter how much it hurt, she was still my mom, and it was the sickness talking, not her. I wanted to be angry at her; after all, the words came from her lips, the decision from her mind and the actions from her body. But even though it looked like her, sounded like her, it wasn't truly her. My LO would never in her right mind say such hurtful ugly words to me. My father asked her to apologize a short while after; but she no longer remembered what she said. She started to deny the whole incident. How could I remain angry? Our emotions are always a choice.

I had to pull myself together and remember that although my feelings are real, they are only indicators not dictators of my actions. While I can't control what life throws at me, I can choose to control how I respond! She is my LO, and I will continue to honor, love and respect her regardless.

While someone else may say, "those words shouldn't hurt you, you know your LO is ill"; even in knowing, the words hurt just as much, and I experienced all types of emotions just the same.

I want to encourage you Today that as we continue to walk along this journey with our LO, while it's ok to feel and process your emotions, don't stay stagnate in what you were meant to overcome.

Father, I need Your help with my emotions. Although I know the truth, I allow words to hurt me just the same. I struggle with the "why" and the lack of understanding. Help me grab ahold of Your sovereignty and accept the fact that I may not ever know the "why"; but I will act with wisdom and love every step of the way. That I may never allow anger, or any negativity drive me to actions not pleasing to You. Please take control of my mind and heart because I trust you! In Jesus' mighty name, AMEN!!

JOURNAL

_____

_____

_____

_____

_____

_____

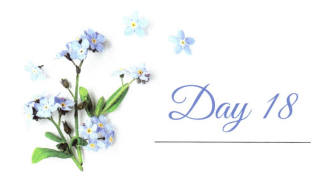

Day 18

Fatigued But Not Surrendered - The ability to continue

Galatians 6:9; James 1:12; Philippians 4:13; John 15:13

>**Galatians 6:9** "Let us not become weary in doing good, for at the proper time we will reap a harvest if we do not give up."
>
>**James 1:12** "Blessed is the man who remains steadfast under trial, for when he has stood the test he will receive the crown of life, which God has promised to those who love him."
>
>**Philippians 4:13** "I can do all things through Him who strengthens me."
>
>**John 15:13** "Greater love has no one than this, that a person will lay down his life for his friends."

<u>Caregiver</u>: A person who serves with empathy and loves you beyond your abilities to do for yourself.

When I took on this task, I never knew how difficult it would be. I never knew how time consuming it would be or how much of me it would demand. I never knew I wouldn't be able to sleep a full night again. I never knew how much it would hurt to see my LO decline. I never knew how desperate I could feel at times. I never knew I would have to reprioritize my life. I never knew I would become a pharmacist, doctor, nurse, accountant, taxi, secretary, administrator, decision maker, maid, assistant, speech therapist, physical therapist, cook, caregiver; all my LO would ever need and remain a daughter, wife, mother, pastor, sibling, mentor, and friend to others.

I never knew how hard life would be without you mom: I never knew how hard it would be to have conversations about how you want things handled once you were gone.

I never knew how hard it would be to watch you fall and not be able to stop you. I never knew how hard it would be to take you from place to place in a wheelchair. I never knew how hard it would be to hear you speak and not make sense. I never knew how hard it would be to convince you to bathe and change clothes. I never knew how much you would argue with me about taking meds. I never knew how hard it would be to watch you suffer through anxiety and depression. I never knew how hard it would be to try and make you understand. I never knew how hard it would be to watch you endure a panic attack. I never knew how hard it would be to repeat myself continuously without you ever understanding. I never knew how hard it would be to stay up with you all night because you couldn't sleep. I never knew how hard it would be to try and get you to do things you once did. I never knew how hard it would be to get you to eat. I never knew how hard it would be to look into your eyes and know you're no longer there. I never knew how hard it would be to accept your anger and not react. I never knew how hard it would be to miss you while you're still present. I never knew how hard it would be to do right by you every day. I never knew how hard it would be to miss you! I never knew how hard it would be to live life with you physically here but not mentally present. I never knew how hard it would be not having our heart to heart talks any longer. I never knew how hard it would be not having a chance to say good-bye. I never knew how hard it would be to mourn you while you're still here. I never knew how lonely it would be. I never knew how hard life would be without you mom.

I'm emotionally, physically and at times spiritually drained but I'm glad I have the privilege of taking care of my LO, I wouldn't have it any other way. Some may look at the glass half empty, but I choose to see it half full.

I will remember for you Mom!

Father, give us strength to continue this journey! We don't know how we are going to make it; but we're glad we have You leading the way. On days we feel lost, remind us that You have us in the palm of Your hands. Please trade our sorrow for joy and give us peace that surpasses all understanding in Jesus' name, Amen!

JOURNAL

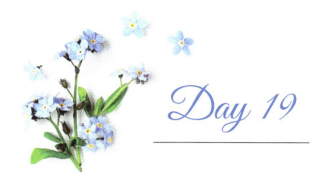

Day 19

Time Management - Time: Once invested you will reap or lose, choose wisely.

Ephesians 5:15-17; Psalm 90:12; Ecclesiastes 3:1

> **Ephesians 5:15-17** "Be very careful, then, how you live—not as unwise but as wise, **16** making the most of every opportunity, because the days are evil. **17** Therefore do not be foolish, but understand what the Lord's will is."
>
> **Psalm 90:12** "Teach us to number our days, that we may gain a heart of wisdom."
>
> **Ecclesiastes 3:1** "There is a time for everything, and a season for every activity under the heavens."

TIME IS ONE OF THE GREATEST GIFTS YOU CAN EVER GIVE, YET SO UNAPPRECIATED.

Time is the one gift that once invested or given, can never be retrieved. Therefore, it's so important that we use it wisely with intention.

We must be wise in the investment of time. Our investment should cause a reciprocal blessing. When we invest time, it should cause us to grow and become better. We must remember that time is extremely valuable because it's so limited.

In whatever capacity you decide to work, you must first invest time in yourself. Whether it's furthering your education, practicing, or exercising, an investment of time is necessary in order for you to provide a service and/or become what you are meant to be. As children, our parents invested time in teaching us the "Do's and Don'ts" while they were teaching us at home how to love, share, eat, walk, and talk; later they sent us to school to learn what we would need to live life as adults. Who we are Today requires an investment of time in order to prepare you. If you think back, you wouldn't be where you are Today without that investment of time. How far we've come or not is all due to the amount of time invested.

In life we are forever learning how to handle things, how to become, even how to handle relationships. No matter what you're doing Today it took an investment of time. When we see the value of time itself, we see the potential in what it has the ability to produce.

In our case, choosing to be a "caregiver" requires us to invest time in ourselves to enable us to serve at our greatest level. You can't pour into someone what you don't have to give. This means that we need to know how to navigate time management. We cannot be the best for others unless we've invested the best in ourselves. We only have the ability to produce after our own kind of what and who we are.

I don't know if you've ever done some gardening or planted anything on your own; but if you have, then you understand that you can't plant an apple tree and expect oranges. You can't sow one thing and reap another. You can only produce what and who you are. Investing time in yourself is not selfish but wise. If you love someone, you must invest time in yourself to be able to give them love. You cannot give what you don't have and what you have requires an investment in yourself, even if it's just to maintain.

Whether you're a caregiver to someone with dementia, Alzheimer or any other disease or impairment, we know it's a 24/7 job. However, it still requires us to be intentional with investing time in ourselves. Your mental health matters! If you are not ok, they are not ok! In my case, I care for both my parents. My mother suffers from dementia but is physically great; while my father's mind is intact but suffers physically from congestive heart failure, kidney disease, liver disease, has a tumor on his kidney, high blood pressure, diabetes, has hemoglobin and iron deficiencies, and requires a monthly paracentesis done at the hospital. Whenever we go out, dad sits in the wheelchair; while I'm pushing the chair I have to hold on to mom because the dementia has caused her to fall several times, once breaking her nose. My day is consumed with giving meds, preparing meals, making phone calls, running errands, making appointments, taking them to where they need to go, and spending time with them; all the while serving my husband, five children, pastoring a church alongside my husband and the list goes on. However, in the beginning I thought I was going to lose my mind. No matter what I did, it wasn't enough. Someone was always complaining or in need and I was just ready to throw in the towel. My stress and anxiety levels were through the roof and I knew I was headed for a mental break down.

I remember wanting to be intentional about spending time with my kids, but it seemed like there wasn't enough hours in the day. So, one morning I heard my daughters leaving the house at 5 a.m. and I asked, "where are you all going?" And they said, "we're headed to the gym" (so yes, you guessed right), as tired as I was, I told them "Hold on, give me five minutes to get ready". I had no idea that I was killing two birds with one stone! Not only was I joining them, but I was releasing stress and soon found myself feeling great emotionally and physically! It cost me some sleep; but it was well worth the investment. I felt like I had hit the jackpot and got a two-for-one blessing!

I soon made that a daily requirement. Although I struggled with exhaustion, I soon mastered it. My parents were going to bed early, around 6:30 p.m. so that gave me the rest of the night to be intentional and invest time in my relationship with my husband and children. You see, everyone around me is important and matters greatly; but I had to be intentional with investing time in myself so I could be my best for them. Its ok to put your needs first! You can never pour out of an empty reservoir! So Today, I challenge you, find that "ME TIME". Whether it's in the AM or late in the PM or perhaps midday. Do something for yourself that causes you to feel fulfilled; whether it's reading, a sport, exercise, or even just taking a ride. Please be intentional. You deserve to be happy and experience your best; and in turn this will allow you to serve them best. You don't have to shortchange yourself to give more, you must invest in yourself to be able to give more. If you value who you are and what you give, you will invest time in yourself!

BE INTENTIONAL, YOU DESERVE IT AND NEED IT.

Father, in the name of Jesus, show us how to value our time and use it wisely. Help us get busy with what has the ability to produce and not with what is wasteful. Allow us to see and understand that investing time in ourselves is not selfish, but necessary. We want to be the best of who You've called us to be and for that we need help with our time. Inspire us and give us creativity to be able to accomplish the task at hand. In your mighty name, Amen!

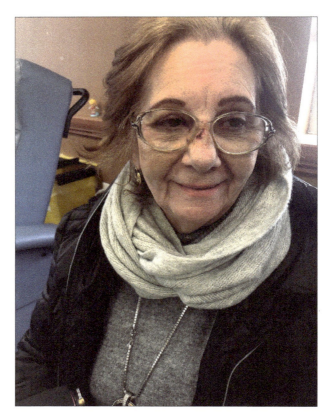

JOURNAL

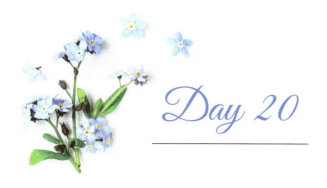

Day 20

Today Great, Tomorrow Who Knows: Sovereignty! Accepting whatever comes even if you don't understand its arrival.

Psalms 115:3; Proverbs 19:21

> **Psalms 115:3** "Our God is in the heavens; he does whatever pleases him."
>
> **Proverbs 19:21** "Many are the plans in a person's heart, but it is the Lord's purpose that prevails."

One of the hardest things I've had to face in this journey is never knowing what the day will bring. The average person can pretty much decide what they will do or perhaps have to face the next day, which affords them the gift of preparation. While a caregiver is always walking in the land of the unknown and unexpected. Daily we travel down the road into the unknown, not knowing what we will have to confront. At times it can be fearful, and at other times debilitating. I've always been a person that loves preparation; I love planning things out strategically. I'm a visionary so this can be overwhelming to say the least. Not having control or a say is so hard. While walking into the unknown, I do the only thing I can do, I dress myself in a strong positive mindset. I grab ahold of unfailing love in preparation for whatever is to come my way. It's almost like a soldier putting on his armor "in case" of a war. Or walking into a minefield carefully, hoping not to set off a bomb. There's no easy way to go about it. All we have to go by is our yesterday; and if yesterday was bad, it give us little room for hope today.

Yesterday my LO called me by my name and told me she loved me. That came accompanied by a great big hug. It felt great to be in her arms and hold her tight. My eyes teared up, I realized right there how much I miss those moments that many take for granted and I didn't want it to end. Today, I told her that I loved her again in hopes of receiving the same reaction from yesterday; but instead she looked at me and said, "ok", her facial expression spoke loud in saying, "I don't know you."

Well, nighttime came, and I went into her room to get her ready for bed. She took her meds, brushed her teeth and was ready to call it a night when she turned to my father and whispered, "who is she?" My heart dropped to my feet, but I couldn't let her see it. My father immediately looked at her and said, "that's Lissette our daughter remember?" Before she could answer, I gave her a big hug and said, "I love you mommy." If her eyes could speak, they would've told me, "But I don't know you." I changed the subject quickly not to make her feel agitated. I looked at her and said, "you're so beautiful mom" she replied, "Thank you." All I can do is hope that tomorrow will be better. I know there's no cure for this horrible plundering disease; but I continue to pray and hope in expectation that things will get better and not worse. I still believe that GOD is a healer so I will place my hope in HIM, the author and finisher of my faith!

God, allow us to see your goodness here in the land of the living. Today, I choose to grab ahold of your faith and declare, "NOW faith is the substance of thing hoped for, the evidence of things not seen." (Hebrews 11:1). While the world is losing hope, I'm grabbing ahold of Your promises. I pray strength for every caregiver reading this that has had to endure this hurtful process. God, it's not easy and its extremely hurtful; but in hindsight it must've been You keeping me and giving me courage all along to endure, so for that, THANK YOU! In Jesus' mighty name, Amen!

JOURNAL

_____

_____

_____

_____

_____

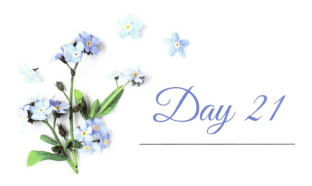

Day 21

Don't Judge Me: Doubt - The feeling of uncertainty at times accompanied by fear.

Luke 6:37; James 4:12; John 8:7

> **Luke 6:37** "Do not judge, and you will not be judged. Do not condemn, and you will not be condemned. Forgive, and you will be forgiven."
>
> **James 4:12** "...But who are you to judge your neighbor?"
>
> **John 8:7** "When they kept on questioning him, he straightened up and said to them, 'Let any one of you who is without sin be the first to throw a stone at her.'"

Life has a way of throwing you some curve balls. It's easy to answer when asked, "what would you do in this situation?" But the truth is you really will never know until you experience it.

For years I prayed that God would render me the opportunity to take care of my parents. I wanted to care for them, watch over them, and serve them. I wanted to spend time with them and get them whatever they would need. I had declared that their last days would be their best!! It was my heart's desire for them. They lived in Florida for 20 years and although I visited often, I missed having them close by. They were now growing older and with all their medical needs, I did not want them to go without. But if I am honest, I didn't know what it would cost me.

I'm a mother of five and when my first three children were born, my parents still lived in NJ. When my last two children were born, my mom came and was even in the delivery room. We've just always been close! My mom was my confidant, my ride-or-die, my mentor, my friend, my ROCK! We were so much alike. There was nothing I wouldn't share with her. Before being diagnosed with dementia, we both agreed when the time came, she would live with me. She made it very known that she wanted to be with me. What a shock when the time approached and I asked her to come but she said, "no!" She wasn't willing to leave her home. One moment she would say, "yes" and the next tell me she never said that.

Well, the day came when it was no longer an option due to unforeseen circumstances. My mother was no longer able to make sound decisions. I asked my father if he was ready to move and He said, "yes." That meant that I had to go to Florida, sell their home and pack up a house full of 20 years worth of memories. I never knew how hard and taxing that would be! I started in November, and It finally came to an end December 6th, 2019! It's amazing how that date still resonates in my heart! I never knew how hard it was going to be to leave that house. It was 20 years worth of unforgettable memories. I considered it my home away from home – my safe place.

I thought once I had them both in NJ it would be a smooth ride; but I soon found out that couldn't be further from the truth. My family struggled with the transition. My husband suggested giving my parents our master bedroom. We lived in a bilevel, and it would've been hard for them to do so many stairs in their medical condition. This left my husband and I sleeping on the floor in the family room for quite some time. Eventually, we bought another mattress and made it our sleeping quarters. But this meant we were invading my children's living space as well. They no longer had a place to come and hang out in, or watch TV, or just relax. Did I mention my dad brought the two dogs he had to join the two dogs I already had? YES, the noise in the house was unbearable. I was the soothing agent between everyone for everything. I felt so bad for my husband and children, but also for my parents. I remember taking a ride down the road of depression. I just took on additional responsibilities to the ones I already had. I was a wife, mother to five, and pastoring alongside my husband. I remember at times I would wait for everyone to be in their rooms at bedtime and I would leave to just cry. I had no space for that at home. My life became so overwhelming. I couldn't see the light at the end of the tunnel. I felt like this move was putting a strain on all my relationships; but what could I do? They are my parents, and this is what I prayed for. In hindsight, sometimes we don't understand why God takes so long to answer our prayers; but now I see that He knew I wasn't ready till that moment and even then I struggled.

I found myself on edge, overwhelmed, frustrated, and no one with whom to share the burden. I knew many looking from the outside in probably thought, "Oh she has a lot of help" but they couldn't be more wrong. I did not want to put this burden on my children or husband. They were my parents, my responsibility, my load. In my thoughts, how could I ask them to help with something in which they had no say. These were my parents and what I prayed for. I just didn't understand that although it was my journey, they would soon be affected by it. It broke my heart to see the look on their face of frustration, anger, and discomfort. They now not only had to share their living space but also my time. I was trying my best to be there as usual, but my other responsibilities became overwhelming. Between doctors' appointments, changing everything over from FL to NJ, looking for a new home, my day-to-day responsibilities, cooking, cleaning, shopping, etc., I literally felt anger. The emotional roller coaster felt like it would never end. On top of everything I was enduring, I had to deal with my LO's breakdowns and anxiety attacks. My father would get upset that I was giving my mother more time and attention. Everything bothered him and he made it known. From comparing my cooking to my mother's, to being picky and making hurtful comments. I just wanted to scream!!!! However, at the same time I tried to understand his frustration too. This was all new to him. He gave up his own home and comfort to get my mother the help she needed. He worked all his life and now had to sacrifice his comfort and way of living. How could I be angry, right? But I was! I just wanted to tell you; you have the right to be angry!! But make sure you have a complete picture of what's causing the anger before moving forward to action. Anger is not the enemy, it's an indication of an emotion letting you know there's something wrong. You can't overcome what you do not accept and confront. Reaction is normally what we do before assessing the situation. Today, I want to challenge you as a caregiver. Although you have the RIGHT to become angry, assess the beginning from the end, find the root and you'll be well on your way to discover your best outcome.

Don't choose the easy way out by just reacting to what's happening, think it through, process it. In understanding, your vision will be transformed.

Father, I need You to help me see things differently. I'm angry in my own right! I didn't sign up for this. This wasn't supposed to turn out this way. I know there has to be another way out; but I'll be honest Lord, I want to quit.

The lack of understanding does that to me. You know I had my heart in the right place; yet here I am, angry, hurt, confused, and frustrated. Please give me eyes to see the truth behind it all and change my perspective in Jesus' mighty name, Amen!

JOURNAL

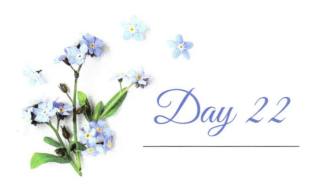

Day 22

Understanding: I Understand You're Not the Same Person Anymore, But I Still Love You

Matthew 7:12; Colossians 4:6; 1 Corinthians 13:4-8

> **Matthew 7:12** "So in everything, do to others what you would have them do to you, for this sums up the Law and the Prophets."

> **Colossians 4:6** "Let your conversation be always full of grace, seasoned with salt, so that you may know how to answer everyone."

> **1 Corinthians 13:4-8** "Love is patient, love is kind. It does not envy, it does not boast, it is not proud. **5** It does not dishonor others, it is not self-seeking, it is not easily angered, it keeps no record of wrongs. **6** Love does not delight in evil but rejoices with the truth. **7** It always protects, always trusts, always hopes, always perseveres. **8** Love never fails. But where there are prophecies, they will cease; where there are tongues, they will be stilled; where there is knowledge, it will pass away."

I never knew it would be possible to miss someone you live with. How can it be possible to miss someone who's still with you? Well, I only know it's possible now, because in being my LO's caregiver, I miss her greatly. I had to come to terms with the reality that she's no longer here, even though I see her body and hear her voice.

I must understand that my LO didn't choose this sickness and disease. She didn't choose to emotionally or mentally be impaired; it was out of her control. When you understand that something out of your control is dominating, then your reaction is different.

When you truly understand a situation, your response and expectations change accordingly.

I love you Mom:

I can't operate in anger when I understand you no longer have the capacity to remember. But with love, and patience, I will continue to remind you.

I can't force you to comprehend by raising my voice or getting frustrated. But with love, and patience I'll continue to echo what you need to hear because I understand.

I can't imagine how confused you must be or how lost you must feel; but I will try my best to reassure you every time, because I love and understand.

I won't lose my patience with you even when you get angry, act out or cry; but I promise to reassure you, because I understand.

When you continue to ask me the same question over and over, I won't yell at you, because I understand.

When I see you're not paying attention or adhering to instructions I won't get angry, because I understand.

When you make mistakes or bad choices I promise not to get upset, because I understand.

Don't worry about forgetting things, I'll be here to remind you, because I understand.

Don't worry if you mess up, I'll be right here to fix it for you, because I understand.

When you've forgotten how to dress yourself, I'll be there to help you, don't worry, because I understand.

When you can no longer comb your hair and get yourself ready, don't worry, I'll do it for you, because I understand.

When you forget how to eat on your own, don't worry I'll feed you, because I understand.

When the time comes and you no longer can do for yourself, don't worry, I'll be here to help you, because I understand.

When you can no longer take a step on your own to walk, don't worry, because I understand.

When you forget my name, I'll lovingly remind you, because I understand.

When you cry in fear, I'll hold you tight, because I understand.

When you start to hallucinate, don't worry, I'll make you feel safe, because I understand.

You won't ever have to face another day alone, I will be with you till the end of time, because I understand.

When you're ready to take your last breath, don't worry, I'll be holding your hand wishing you could stay, but I understand.

Even now you're teaching me how to love because I understand.

I love you Mom!

Father, first I want to thank you for giving me the best mother I could've ever had. She showed me what it was to love unconditionally. I guess she learned that from You.

There's nothing she wouldn't have given or sacrificed for me growing up. So now I want to give it back to her. Please help me be the best possible gift for her life. I pray that You would fill me with love, patience, and joy as I serve her.

Bring healing to her mind and help her feel Your love and peace along the way in Jesus' mighty name, AMEN!!

JOURNAL

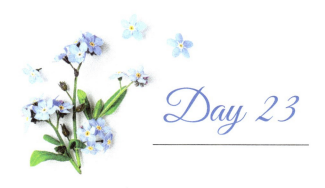

Day 23

**Determined: Having made a firm unchangeable decision.
I Will Love You Till The End**

1 Corinthians 16:14; Colossians 3:14; John 15:13

1 Corinthians 16:14 "Do everything in love."

Colossians 3:14 "And over all these virtues put on love, which binds them all together in perfect unity."

John 15:13 "Greater love has no one than this, that someone lay down his life for his friends."

Mom, I'm determined to make your last days be your best days:

I can't imagine what life was like for you when you arrived here from Puerto Rico. You didn't know the language or lifestyle, yet you took on the challenge. You made this new land your home to give your children a greater chance at a better life.

I can't imagine how hard it must've been for you to get your driver's license and work in a factory with all the impossibilities facing you daily. No matter what came your way, you were resilient and determined to make it. From fear, to false promises, to not having the comfort or support of your parents, nothing stopped you or Dad. You both created a plan and with time and determination you made it!

You were both hard workers all your lives. I remember at times you would stay home to take care of us; but when things were tight, you got dressed and went back to work. No matter how much you hustled you were always there for your family. I remember you would make my clothes and dresses. You always had us looking rich even when we didn't have a dime to our name. No matter what, we never went without.

I remember the first home you and dad purchased; I was only three years old. That soon became my safe haven till I left to get married twenty years later. I remember the gardens you planted yourself. Some with flowers and others with plants and herbs. When I was sick, you would go into your garden and pick some leaves from your mint plant. You would boil it and give me tea to settle my stomach. You were so intentional and great at all you did.

You were the best mother, greatest example, best role model, greatest mentor, loving, kind, generous, and the best teacher of all. You have well equipped me for life. The one and only thing you never did was prepare me for your departure. I know you use to always say, "I need you to learn this because I'm not always going to be around" and I would reply, "Yes you are!" I didn't understand then what I well understand now.

Your father took you from your mother when you were only five. He gave you a stepmother you never asked for, who treated you like a slave. At the tender age of nine, they took you out of school so you could become a babysitter to your half brothers and sisters, maid, cook, errand runner, animal feeder, and human laundry mat for your siblings, family, and stepmothers' sisters. You suffered at such a tender age. I guess that's why you were determined to give me and my siblings the best life possible. Now I understand why you said, "I need you to learn because I'm not always going to be around" you were determined to give your children the best life possible. You wanted us to be well prepared. So now I'm returning the favor. I'm determined that your last days will be your best days. Yes, it's coming at a cost; but looking back its so well worth it.

Mom, even with dementia I'll love and take care of you. Even as you continue to drift away, I'll love and take care of you. Until the good Lord calls you home, I will love and take care of you. You did right by me and my siblings and even your grandchildren, now I will do right by you.

I love you with all my heart and forever! I am who I am Today because of who you were yesterday!

Father, grant me the strength I need in suffering such a great loss. Help me to have the ability to give back all she gave and poured into me with interest! Use me to bless her whole life. I'm willing to be Your hands, Your heart, and Your feet here on earth. You gave me the best when You gave her to me, help me be the same. I love You and thank You for Mom being such an unforgettable great gift of life.

In Jesus' name, Amen!

JOURNAL

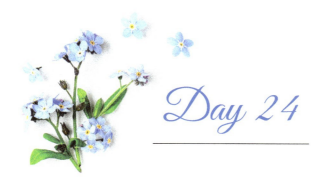

Day 24

Ambiguous Mourning: Accepting and Mourning Those Who Have Not Yet Departed

Matthew 5:4; Revelation 21:4; Psalms 116:15

Matthew 5:4 "Blessed are those who mourn, for they shall be comforted."

Revelation 21:4 "He will wipe away every tear from their eyes, and death shall be no more, neither shall there be mourning, nor crying, nor pain anymore, for the former things have passed away."

Psalms 116:15 "Precious in the sight of the Lord is the death of his saints."

How do we accept the new, without fully understanding how and exactly when we lost the old? I was told that we mourn those who have died and are no longer with us. We cry and grieve for them. We even wear black clothing as an expression of grief. But no one has explained how to mourn for someone who's still physically here. This is a whole different level of loss, pain and grief. There's no set date for their departure. The loss is gradual and subtle, which I believe makes it harder to accept.

When we lose someone we love, we all endure the process of pain and grief; however, they are different for everyone. In the evidence of the suffered loss, we can cope with what we're facing because the loss is not hidden from our eyes. However, I believe the pain is greater when the loss is invisible. I've now come to understand that mourning someone who is still alive is very possible and excruciating.

When we mourn the loss of a LO we're surrounded by others and are comforted by their words, actions, and presence. We somehow find closure, despite the pain we're confronting. However, an ambiguous loss is completely different. Closure is nowhere in sight and the lack of understanding often results in unresolved grief. No one is there to support or help you walk this journey because there's no acknowledgement of the same. No one notices the loss you're suffering because it's not superficial. If undetected, we will walk into a place of greater pain leading us into isolation.

Not identifying your feelings and/or emotions can cause an extensive amount of turmoil in your life. It has the potential to harm you, not only mentally, but physically.

When you're so busy taking care of your LO and every day is an unexpected new adventure, you must be intentional with the following:

- A) Take time to identify and acknowledge what you're feeling.

Allow yourself to feel and grieve. An imposter has taken over your LO's body.

- B) Never let go of memories; but cherish them while trying to create new ones.

- C) Accept the new person they have become and love them through it. Remember this wasn't a choice for them.

- D) Take care of yourself and be intentional about it. You can only give your best when you're at your best.

- E) Its ok to ask for help! You're not alone. Explaining to others may furnish you the ability to receive help.

Father, I'm in so much pain. I'm grieving my LO even though they're physically still here. Please don't misunderstand me. I'm grateful to have my LO; but I miss her dearly at the same time. Can You give me peace and help me endure my loss? I want to be able to still love her through this transition. I don't know her anymore. I know she didn't choose this, but neither did I. Help me serve her and do it well as unto You. Allow me to feel Your love in me exude through me. In Jesus' mighty name, AMEN!

JOURNAL

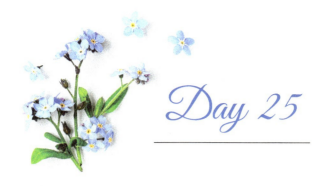

Day 25

Confidence: Your Love Has Taught Me Well!

2 Timothy 1:5; Proverbs 22:6; Philippians 1:3

> **2 Timothy 1:5** "I am reminded of your sincere faith, a faith that dwelt first in your grandmother Lois and your mother Eunice and now, I am sure, dwells in you as well."

> **Proverbs 22:6** "Train up a child in the way he should go; even when he is old he will not depart from it."

> **Philippians 1:3** "I thank my God in all my remembrance of you"

Mom: Every day when I look in the mirror, I'm reminded of you! I see part of you in me. While I'm trying to embody everything you were, I thank God for what I already see.

I am who I am Today because of what you imparted in me. You loved me enough to correct me when I was wrong, direct me when I was lost, your words healed me when I was hurt, you loved me enough to embrace me with all my faults, your love carried me when I couldn't move forward, your love paved the way for my future.

One thing I was certain about all my life was your love! I felt like there was nothing I couldn't face or overcome because your love would always be there. It built such a great confidence in me that even now it affords me the ability to care for you when you most need it.

One thing I want you to know is that I will be ok because of you! In the moments you've come back mentally not only can I tell by the look in your eyes; but also by your words of concern. The last time this happened, it was your birthday June 25th, 2021. You looked at me in the eyes with a look of terror, crying and saying, "Lissette, this isn't what I wanted for you, I'm so sorry Lissette." Then you slipped away again. I knew it was you because you never call me by my name. I tried to reassure you before you left; but not sure I was able to accomplish that. Although it's not what you wanted for me, I want you to know that you're safe. Have confidence in what you built in me. My desire is to become all of who you were and all you represented. I love you so much Mom. Thank you, because Today, I am strong, and I walk in confidence because of you.

Today, I want to encourage the reader to be confident in who you already are! I know this journey doesn't come with a road map or instructions; but the mere fact that you're trying makes you a winner! Look at yourself in the mirror and remind yourself how great you are. Not everyone can do what you're doing! Knowledge is power, so remind yourself and build your self-confidence daily. I believe in you, you're stronger than you think!

Father, thank You for revealing your strength in us. Please continue to reassure us that we have what it takes to continue down this journey. Build our confidence in You daily. We know we can't do this without You so thank you for choosing us, for such a meaningful task. Continue to guide and lead us every day. While some days are easier than others, I trust and I'm confident in Your power and love, Amen!

JOURNAL

_____

_____

_____

_____

_____

_____

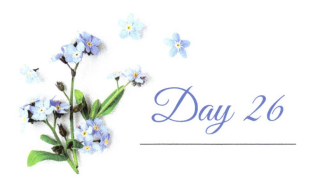

Day 26

I Have Rights: I Have Feelings Too!

Colossians 4:6; Matthew 11:28; Hebrews 12:15; Isaiah 55:9

> **Colossians 4:6** "Let your conversation be always full of grace, seasoned with salt, so that you may know how to answer everyone."

> **Matthew 11:28** "Come to me, all you who are weary and burdened, and I will give you rest."

> **Hebrews 12:15** "See to it that no one falls short of the grace of God and that no bitter root grows up to cause trouble and defile many."

> **Isaiah 55:9** "For as the heavens are higher than the earth, so are my ways higher than your ways and my thoughts than your thoughts."

If I'm going to be honest, my feelings do matter! I have a husband and children to care for. In being a caregiver to my LO's it doesn't mean that I abandon my responsibilities to my husband and children; it just means I must reorganize my time to best serve everyone I love, including myself. I must understand that there's only twenty-four hours in a day and only so much can be accomplished; however; I need the ability to prioritize so no one lacks or struggles. I'll admit in the beginning it was extremely hard for me. Everything seemed to be top priority and I felt like all the work fell on my shoulders to figure out. However, now I'm better and seem to have it all under control. I made adjustments that helped everyone to feel loved and cared for.

I have four siblings. Three brothers that live out of state, and one of them has been MIA (missing in action) for almost two years, no phone call, or any way of reaching him, by his own choice. I've tried several ways of reaching out to him with no avail. I just don't understand why he wouldn't want to speak or be concerned about his parents. Especially when he knows their time is limited. My sister, who is the eldest lives an hour away and comes to visit when possible, but calls daily. That leaves me, I'm the youngest of the five siblings. If I'm honest, I chose this; but I didn't know how hard it would be. The only thing I was certain of was that it was the right thing to do for my parents!

I was sure that my LO's family would call and check on her; but that has been infrequent so far. Most of the time I initiate the contact. After the diagnosis, I came to learn quickly that people who were once close family and friends, now are nowhere to be found. I'm certain they will be the same ones showing up for the funeral and making a performance. While I hope I'm wrong, time will tell.

Although my mother is now suffering from dementia and probably won't remember everyone, that doesn't give them the right to forget she ever existed. She may not remember them; but those caring for her and living with her will remember their absence in her time of need. Real love doesn't leave at the sign of a disease, that's when it truly should manifest.

They don't know how hard it is to watch the decline day by day, because they've chosen to stay away. They don't know what she needs because they are not around to see. They have no idea how much she misses them, because they haven't been concerned enough to check. It's sad that they will come to honor her on her death bed; but not in life while they still have a chance. It makes me angry that they think it's ok to abandon her in her time of sickness, while they go on with day-to-day life. Her mind may be wasting away; but mine is strong and taking notes.

To those family members I say: forgive me in advance if I don't run and throw my arms around you to show you love. I'm too busy mourning two losses – my LO's and your relationship that no longer exists. The truth hurts; but I have the right to share these feelings you set into motion. While I refuse to waste my energy on hate, I still thought you should know - I have rights too!

Father, I need Your help. While I continue to deal with my LO's decline, help me to deal with my heart. Don't allow bitterness or resentment to take root, that's not what I'm looking for, but I hurt. Thank You for understanding me and given me the strength to endure. Had it not been for You I don't know where I would be. Help me not harbor offense and continue to show love despite of circumstances. In Jesus' mighty name! Amen.

JOURNAL

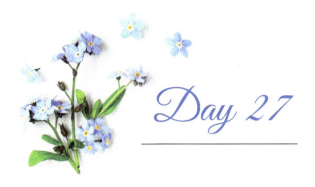

Day 27

Memories: I Miss Who You Used to Be

1 John 4:19; Proverbs 23:22; Ephesians 6:1-3

1 John 4:19 "We love because he first loved us."

Proverbs 23:22 "Listen to your father who gave you life, and do not despise your mother when she is old."

Ephesians 6:1-3 "Children, obey your parents in the Lord, for this is right. **2** 'Honor your father and mother'—which is the first commandment with a promise— **3** 'so that it may go well with you and that you may enjoy long life on the earth.'"

My LO was such an active person. She was always doing something. Whether it was cooking, cleaning, fixing something, sewing, gardening, etc. I never really saw her sitting down. Even while she was eating, she would stand. It was almost like she was constantly racing against the clock.

She helped my father pastor a church for many years. She would preach, teach, give counsel, mentor, even drive the church van to pick people up for service. She was always willing to serve others. She was so full of life and giving.

I miss the way she used to cook. Her food was like no other. When I wanted to learn how to cook, I would ask, "so how much salt do you add?" and she would say, "more or less" (in Spanish "mas o menos"). I would ask again for the next ingredient, and she would give me the same answer. I would laugh so hard and say, "mom, how am I supposed to learn?" And she replied, "by looking and paying attention" she never used measurements in her life. That's the way it was for everything. No matter what she put her hands to, she mastered it. She started cooking at the age of nine for a family of twelve so she had plenty of experience. Now every time one of my children ask me how to cook something and want exact quantities, I reply the same way!

I miss seeing her glow. She was so full of life. I miss our daily phone calls. At times we would call each other two or three times a day. Even when I traveled to other countries for my job, she would come and stay with my children. She never missed a beat and always knew when something was wrong. I miss her wisdom and counsel. She taught me so much, not only by what she said but by how she lived. She is truly the Proverbs 31 ("The Wife of Noble Character") woman.

Now I'm making new memories while missing the old ones. I will be forever grateful for every lesson learned, for every correction, for every word of wisdom, and for every moment in her life! She's made me better in every way. So today, while I'm missing her, I choose to enjoy every moment left, for I have come to understand what a true gift it is.

Father, I just want to thank You for what once was but also for what now is. I'm grateful for her life. For every part of my life, she was always there. Please help me remember that she never failed me so that I can continue to try and live up to that. Help me live the rest of my days trying to make her proud whether she remembers or not. Thank You for blessing me with the gift of her life, in Jesus' name, Amen!

JOURNAL

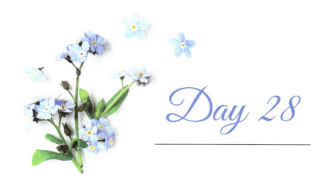

Day 28

FEAR: Can I Really Do This?

Isaiah 41:10; 2 Timothy 1:7; 1 John 4:18; Psalm 34:4

> **Isaiah 41:10** "So do not fear, for I am with you; do not be dismayed, for I am your God. I will strengthen you and help you; I will uphold you with my righteous right hand."
>
> **2 Timothy 1:7** "For the Spirit God gave us does not make us timid, but gives us power, love and self-discipline."
>
> **1 John 4:18** "There is no fear in love. But perfect love drives out fear, because fear has to do with punishment. The one who fears is not made perfect in love."
>
> **Psalm 34:4** "I sought the Lord, and he answered me; he delivered me from all my fears."

When things don't go your way, it's not an indication of failure. No matter how much planning we do or how much preparation goes into your day, it doesn't mean it's going to work out that way. You may have the greatest intentions in the world; but unfortunately, we don't control the outcome.

I remember for my LO's birthday we had great plans! We decided that everyone was going to take the day off from work including my sister that lives an hour away and we were going to celebrate mom. If there's one thing this pandemic proved, it was that life is too short. I had ordered a specialty cake; made reservations and we had the whole day planned out.

We all woke up with great expectations that day for all we had planned. As I was serving my parents breakfast and getting their coffee, I started to tell them about the plans of the day with great enthusiasm. We had decorated the house the night before with balloons, streamers, a "Happy Birthday" banner, and roses. She always loved roses.

After breakfast, I wanted to bathe her and get her pretty for her celebration. Suddenly, she started arguing, she was not going to bathe. She argued that she was clean. I gave in and said, "okay, well let's just change into your new clothes." That didn't work either. We thought of every little detail possible and so far, it wasn't going as planned.

I thought for sure when my sister arrived, my LO would change her mind and attitude, but that wasn't the case. My LO started to cry and go down the path of a meltdown. Meanwhile, I was stressed because my children and husband had taken the day off to celebrate her. They all started asking what we were going to do. Again, I started to stress thinking, "I hate to think they took the day off for nothing" emotions where running high and everyone looked to me for answers, including my dad.

I have medication to calm her down; but I don't like medicating her unless it's beyond my ability to talk her out of it. Well, that was the day out of all days! I felt like such a failure. Everyone around me was asking what we were doing. Rightfully so! They took the day off, we had plans, now what? I went next to her in bed and did the only thing I knew how to, I laid hands on her and began to pray for God's peace over her mind and life. All of a sudden, she started crying out to God as well. With tears streaming down her face, she started to say, "God help me, I don't want to feel like this." I opened my eyes and just looked at her. What she was praying actually made sense. She continued to cry out and pray and I did the same. After a few minutes I wiped her tears and tried to console her. She looked in my eyes and said, "Lissette, I'm so sorry, this isn't what I wanted for you"; struggling to hold back my tears and comforting her, I looked at her and said, "Mom?" And she replied, "yes." For a moment she gave me a gift on her birthday! It was her, the real her, the old her, the one I missed dearly! I affirmed her and reassured her that it was a privilege for me to take care of her and that I loved her so much; but instantly she disappeared again.

This journey is such an unexpected emotional roller coaster. The unknown always has the ability to cause fear; but remember you're doing a great job and you have what it takes! Every situation we encounter is just knowledge we're obtaining as we go along the way. Its wisdom and revelation that you may need to use later down the road; but at the very least, it is a blessing to share with others. Whatever you do, don't allow fear to arrest you and make you quit! Remember, F.E.A.R. is False Evidence Appearing Real! You CAN do this! YOU have what it takes! Just let God lead the way!

Father, in moments unknown help me to remember that I can face whatever comes before me. Give me wisdom and strategies to help me down this path. Allow me to be the voice of reason and encouragement to others. If You can do it for me, you can do it for them. In Jesus' mighty name, Amen!

JOURNAL

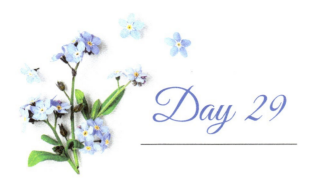

Day 29

Anxiety - Intense, excessive, and persistent worry and fear about everyday situations.

1 Peter 5:7; Matthew 6:34

1 Peter 5:7 "casting all your anxieties on him, because he cares for you."

Matthew 6:34 "Therefore do not be anxious about tomorrow, for tomorrow will be anxious for itself. Sufficient for the day is its own trouble."

If you're a caregiver, then you've experience anxiety at one time or another. Perhaps more than most. The unknown elements of this illness can be mortifying. In my case, I had to learn to think ahead of what could happen in order to take preventive measures. At times, I feel like my mind just can't shut down. I feel like I have to always be ahead of the situation. Unfortunately, my efforts aren't enough at times, she fell yet again looking straight at me. Her face hit the ground first causing her to bruise her cheek bone, arm, and leg. My LO no longer has the ability to brace herself when falling. I felt so horrible, she fell again while being with me.

When this took place, my anxiety shot through the roof! How could this happen? My heart broke as she tried to explain to me how she didn't understand what happened. The look of terror and fear in her eyes was paralyzing. I hugged her and tried to comfort her as best as I could.

Anxiety started to take a toll on me and now it was joining force with guilt. I was emotionally, mentally, and physically drained all the time. I found it hard to sleep, always anxious. I actually have a baby monitor on my night table to listen to my mother and father at night. I've become a light sleeper; I hear everything now and during the day I have a camera in their room and one in the kitchen for when I run errands. Although she is never left alone, I would go out and look at the cameras in the house every two or three minutes. I couldn't be away and at peace.

I finally took a vacation with my husband. My sister and adult children stayed in the house with my LO and Father. Even being away and knowing they were in good hands, I would still check in often, look at the cameras and call, I just couldn't disconnect. While I was away, I remember having a dream that my LO passed away and I wasn't there. I literally woke up crying hysterically. My husband had to calm me down and remind me it was only a dream.

I guess what I'm trying to say is that if you're not being intentional, anxiety will wreak havoc on you! Finally, I had to pray and ask God for peace. I remember I took a walk on the beach and just prayed and prayed. I gave God all my concerns and worries. As I walked back to the hotel, a weight lifted. Sometimes we're carrying loads that weren't meant for us to carry. Yes, I believe this could be your God given assignment; but it's not supposed to wear you down. That's never God's intention. I soon remembered what 1 Peter 5:7 says: "casting all your anxieties on him, because he cares for you." It's truly that simple! God heard my prayer while at the beach, and I walked away feeling uplifted.

I want to encourage you; whatever you're feeling and going through HE cares! You have nothing to lose but a lot of peace to gain. God has a great track record, why do I say this? David must've been enduring hard times when he wrote Psalm 27:13-14. I will paraphrase: "I would have lost heart unless I had believed that I would see the goodness of the Lord in the land of the living: Wait on the Lord; be of good courage, and He shall strengthen your heart, wait, I say, on the Lord!"

So, I have decided to wait on the Lord and break up with anxiety! We haven't been good for each other! I hope you consider joining me! Never hold on to something that hasn't been good to you!

Father, help me continue to wait on You. At times it's so hard and I feel like I get consumed with what's happening at the moment. Remind me that waiting on You will cause me to hold on to hope in times of anxiety. Don't allow anxiety to rule my heart, mind, and soul. Today, I'm giving You all that I am, for all that You are! In Jesus' mighty name, Amen!

JOURNAL

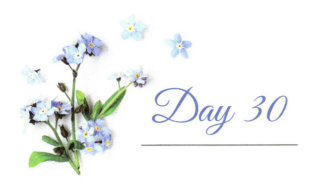

Day 30

My Assignment - A task entrusted and assigned to me.

Jeremiah 29:11; Ephesians 2:10

> **Jeremiah 29:11** "For I know the plans I have for you," declares the Lord, "plans to prosper you and not to harm you, plans to give you hope and a future."

> **Ephesians 2:10** "For we are his workmanship, created in Christ Jesus for good works, which God prepared beforehand, that we should walk in them."

In life we eventually come to a point where we search for purpose. We start to ask questions like, "why am I here?" "What good am I?" "Will I ever accomplish anything?" Some of us continue our education and others may pursue a trade; but it all leads back to the same – seeking fulfillment.

As believers, we search for the will of God in our lives. Everyone ultimately seeks fulfillment, and fulfillment is only found in completing our assignment. Have you ever started a project and actually finished it? The feeling of satisfaction is so gratifying, we feel fulfilled until our next assignment.

Have you ever asked yourself questions like, "why me?" "I don't know if I can do this." "Can I do this?" 'What am I doing?" "Why do I even care?" Perhaps everything that has transpired is proving to you that this is your assignment. Despite what you may see or think, despite what others have said, God has a way of giving us assignments that allow us to be our best and be blessed. If you know God, then you know He's intentional.

Everything we go through in life is not only for us, but for others. If my experiences can help someone else, then those experiences were well worth the struggle. At times when I feel like a failure, I'm reminded that great people weren't born great, they failed time and time again to become great.

On this journey, we're bound to fail at times; but it doesn't mean we weren't called to this or assigned to it. It simply means we're learning to become. With all my fears, failures, hurt, anger, frustration, and bewilderment, my hope is to help others succeed where I failed. If I can accomplish this, the blessing will be reciprocal.

I know the cost associated with this journey all too well; and while I don't understand it fully, I grab ahold of God's sovereignty.

If this is my life's assignment, I want to hear Him say, "well done!"

There will be no greater accomplishment!

Father, thank You for trusting me for this assignment. In Your divinity, You could've chosen anyone else, but You chose and equipped me for the same. Help us to understand Your purpose and will. Give us eyes to see what You see and give us wisdom and understanding to endure. In Jesus' mighty name, Amen!

JOURNAL

_____

_____

_____

_____

_____

_____

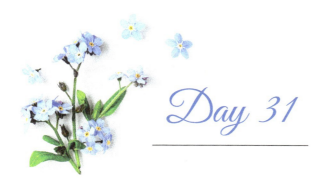

Day 31

Until Then - I'm willing to give you my best, despite the sacrifice!

Ephesians 5:15-17; Colossians 4:5; Philippians 1:6

> **Ephesians 5:15-17** "Be very careful, then, how you live—not as unwise but as wise, **16** making the most of every opportunity, because the days are evil. **17** Therefore do not be foolish, but understand what the Lord's will is."
>
> **Colossians 4:5** "Be wise in the way you act toward outsiders; make the most of every opportunity."
>
> **Philippians 1:6** "being confident of this, that he who began a good work in you will carry it on to completion until the day of Christ Jesus."

There's one thing I'm sure, when we're expectant, we tend to be well prepared. We find ourselves preparing for what's to come, whether good or bad. Even when we don't know exactly how or when it will come, we can still make time to prepare. While we're waiting, we can become intentional with our actions and time.

When my LO was first diagnosed with dementia, it was hard for me to grasp.

While the diagnosis rocked my world, I chose to make every minute count.

The only way I could accomplish this was by putting my LO first. In putting someone first, whether out of love, empathy, concern, or desperation, it comes with a price. Most of the time we will pay the cost for the value we see in it.

At the present moment, the only thing that matters is time. Not knowing how much of it I have left to spend with my LO pushes me to sacrifice whatever is necessary. Time is the only thing we can't buy, but we can invest it.

As I write this even now, I'm still unaware of the time I have left with my LO; but I do my best to make every moment meaningful. Many times, we're sacrificing something we like or prefer to make a moment with our LO count. In doing so, please remember this will not always be the case. Time is not on our side. The day will come when your LO transitions and you no longer can sacrifice. I know it's hard at times, it can even cause anger, resentment, or frustration at the moment; but this too shall pass. This hardship will not last forever.... read that again: This hardship will not last forever! I know at times it feels like forever. We see others moving on with life and it feels like ours has stopped. We've lost friends, family and at times even spouses; but I want to encourage you, you're doing the right thing. How can I possibly know that? Because you're doing what's necessary and what no one else could or wanted to do. Sure, it's easy for others to talk because they're not doing it. It's easy for others to criticize or complain because they're not doing it. It's even easy for others to give their opinion while they're not the ones sacrificing; but don't spend your time on those things, remember – our time is limited. Be intentional on how you spend your time. Time is an unrecognized gift that's limited.

On special holidays I can't help but think, will this be the last one? It brings sadness, but at the same time intentionality. It brings me back to the beginning. I don't know how many years, months, days, weeks, or hours I have left so I choose to be intentional every minute of every day.

Are you looking for the truth? The truth is that the future holds nothing good for us. No matter how much we do or not, the outcome will be the same. We are all facing the inevitable. Our LO's final day will come; but when it does, will you have any regrets? I'd rather live a time of sacrifice than a life of regret. So, I will be intentional in making the best of everyday, until whatever is going to happen, happens. We may not be able to stop it from happening; but we can determine how we will handle it.

I want to encourage you to start over! Today is a new day! Be Intentional, be purposeful, be wise and most of all be loving to your LO as if they were still the same as when you first loved them.

There's nothing wrong with starting over. As a matter of fact, it's prudent!

A new month is about to begin, so go back to day one and let's start again!

Mom your dementia won't stop me.

Dad your medical needs can't stop me.

Father, Thank You for always giving me exactly what I've needed. In hindsight, I see You every step of the way, even when I couldn't see or feel You at the time. Your love has carried me through some of the hardest times. In times of insecurity and frustration, You always made a way and reassured me. I don't know where I would be without You so, please continue to guide and lead me, I love You!

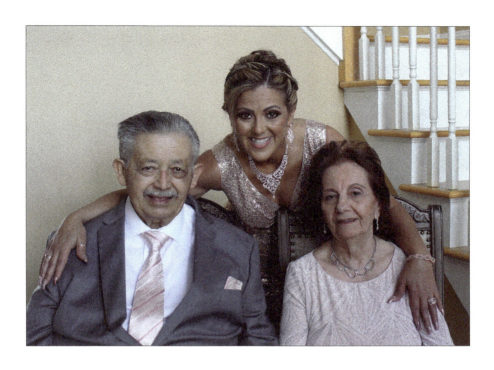

JOURNAL

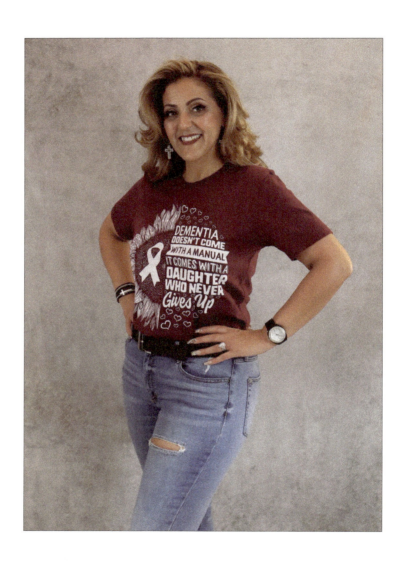

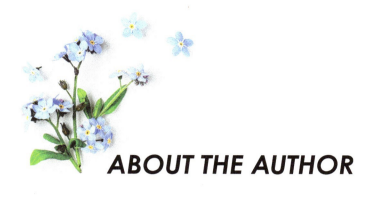

ABOUT THE AUTHOR

*P*astor Lissette Rodriguez is the co-founder and lead pastor along with her husband Elijah Rodriguez of Hope Worship Center in Aberdeen, New Jersey. She preaches and teaches God's infallible word with passion and is committed to building others while establishing God's kingdom.

She's an amazing wife to Elijah Rodriguez and mother of five children: Jeremiah, Vanessa, Leah, Rebecca, and Marcus. The last few years she has become a dedicated caregiver to her loving parents Emilio and Crucita Negron.

You can follow her on instagram at: pastor_liz_rodriguez or email her at: pastorlissette@hopewc.org

CPSIA information can be obtained
at www.ICGtesting.com
Printed in the USA
BVHW021203310822
645866BV00019B/294